CLINICAL MANUAL OF OTOLARYNGOLOGY

NOTICE

Medicine is an ever-changing science. As new research and clinical experience broaden our knowledge, changes in treatment and drug therapy are required. The author and the publisher of this work have checked with sources believed to be reliable in their efforts to provide information that is complete and generally in accord with the standards accepted at the time of publication. However, in view of the possibility of human error or changes in medical sciences, neither the author nor the publisher nor any other party who has been involved in the preparation or publication of this work warrants that the information contained herein is in every respect accurate or complete, and they are not responsible for any errors or omissions or for the results obtained from use of such information. Readers are encouraged to confirm the information contained herein with other sources. For example and in particular, readers are advised to check the product information sheet included in the package of each drug they plan to administer to be certain that the information contained in this book is accurate and that changes have not been made in the recommended dose or in the contraindications for administration. This recommendation is of particular importance in connection with new or infrequently used drugs.

CLINICAL MANUAL OF OTOLARYNGOLOGY

SECOND EDITION

Terence M. Davidson, M.D., F.A.C.S.

Professor of Otolaryngology—Head and Neck Surgery
Associate Dean for Continuing Medical Education
University of California Medical School and
Veterans Administration Medical Center
San Diego, California

McGraw-Hill, Inc.
Health Professions Division

New York   St. Louis   San Francisco   Auckland
Bogotá   Caracas   Lisbon   London   Madrid
Mexico   Milan   Montreal   New Delhi
Paris   San Juan   Singapore   Sydney   Tokyo   Toronto

CLINICAL MANUAL OF OTOLARYNGOLOGY

1234567890   HAL HAL   98765432

ISBN 0-07-105399-9

This book was set in Times Roman by J.M. Post Graphics, Corp.
The editors were Michael J. Houston and Lester A. Sheinis;
the production supervisor was Richard C. Ruzycka;
the project supervision was by Tage Publishing Service, Inc.;
the cover designer was Marsha Cohen/Parallelogram;
Arcata Graphics/Halliday was printer and binder.

Library of Congress Cataloging-in-Publication Data

Davidson, Terence M.
  Clinical manual of otolaryngology.

    Rev. ed. of: Manual of otolaryngology—head and
neck surgery. © 1984.
    Includes bibliographical references and index.
    1. Otolaryngology—Handbooks, manuals, etc.
2. Head—Surgery—Handbooks, manuals, etc.   3. Neck
Surgery—Handbooks, manuals, etc.   I. Davidson,
Terence M. Manual of otolaryngology—head and neck
surgery. II. Title. [DNLM: 1. Head—surgery.
2. Neck—Surgery.   WE 705 / D253m]
RF56.D39 1992   617.5′1   91-3857
ISBN 0-07-105399-9 (softcover)

Contents

Preface

Most medical students today spend a total of 2 weeks or less on an otolaryngology—head and neck surgery—rotation, yet anywhere from 30 to 50 percent of patients presenting to primary care physicians have complaints referable to the head and neck. Most of the textbooks on otolaryngology are long, too detailed, and contain more basic science than medical students and primary care providers require to diagnose and treat the majority of otolaryngology diseases. This book is concise, practical, and readable.

Otolaryngology is an old field formerly called Ear, Nose, and Throat (ENT). It now encompasses general otolaryngology (diseases of the ear, nose, and throat), neurotology, head and neck cancer, and facial plastic and reconstructive surgery. Some call the field otolaryngology and others call it otolaryngology—head and neck surgery.

The goal of this book is to describe only the most common and important diseases in otolaryngology—head and neck surgery. A simple, straightforward approach is used. Esoteric physiology, anatomy, and pharmacology, as well as the uncommon diseases, are excluded. Selected case presentations and differential diagnoses are presented to help unite pertinent information. All physicians should be able to diagnose the maladies described here. They should then be able to treat or properly refer a patient for treatment.

The outline from which this book was created was developed for the otolaryngology—head and neck surgery medical student rotation at the University of California at San Diego. Because it has been found so useful by our students, it is included as an appendix at the end of this book.

The physical examination involved in otolaryngology can only be learned from an otolaryngologist. It cannot be learned by reading this or any other text. By the same token, procedures such as controlling epistaxis, suturing, and performing a tracheostomy can only be learned by observing the procedures and then performing them under supervision. Videotapes to assist in these endeavors can be obtained through the American Academy of Otolaryngology–Head and Neck Surgery or through the Department of Otolaryngology–Head and Neck Surgery at the University of California Medical School, San Diego.

If additional knowledge of this field is wanted, more detailed textbooks are listed at the end of the text. In addition, the most recent information can be found in journal articles.

I hope you enjoy reading this manual, for I enjoyed writing it. If you have any questions, ask them. If you have any constructive comments, write me a letter. I will appreciate it. Good luck to you.

Acknowledgments

My special thanks go to Dr. Alan Nahum, for teaching me head and neck surgery and for helping me organize it for this text. I thank my father, Dr. Norman Davidson, for giving me a start a long time ago, helping me along the way, and assisting me in the presentation of this material. I am deeply indebted to my third-year medical students, for they have taught me what they wanted to learn, and have been invaluable in improving this text. My closest friends and supporters in this endeavor have been my children, Daniel and Benjamin, who have inspired and encouraged me in this project.

I also appreciate the advice and direction provided by my colleagues, the faculty at UCSD, with special recognition to Dr. Roberta Cueva for rewriting the otology chapter and Dr. Thomas Robbins for improvements in the head and neck cancer chapter.

CLINICAL MANUAL OF OTOLARYNGOLOGY

CHAPTER 1

Head and Neck History and Physical Examination

The head and neck examination is complex. It is best learned by demonstration and practice under the guidance of an experienced clinician.

REVIEW OF SYSTEMS

The following is a basic review of systems. Any positive findings should be investigated thoroughly.

SKIN: Do you have any skin tumors, sores, or black pigmented moles?

EYES: Do you have any problems with your eyes? Any problems seeing? Do you wear glasses? Do you have any pain or infection? Do your eyes dry out or tear? Do your eyes itch?

EARS: Do you have or have you ever had any decrease in hearing? Do you have ringing in your ears? Have you ever had ear infections, drainage, or surgery? Do you have any ear pain? Do you have any trouble with balance or dizziness?

NOSE: Do you have any trouble breathing through your nose? Do you ever have bleeding or clear or cloudy drainage from your nose? Have you any problems smelling or tasting foods? Any problems with sinus infections or an itchy nose?

MOUTH: Do you have any problems in your mouth with sores, tooth infections, sore throats, or unusual pain? Have you had your tonsils or adenoids removed?

THROAT: Do you have any problems swallowing? Any trouble breathing, speaking, or coughing? Have you experienced any voice changes? Any lumps or pains in your neck? Do you have a history of irradiation to your neck or throat? (Problems relating to the thyroid are covered under the endocrine review of systems.)

PHYSICAL EXAMINATION

Examination of the Skin

The skin should be inspected and the scalp palpated for sores or tumors. Basal cell and epidermoid tumors are looked for, as well as pigmented lesions suspicious for melanoma.

Examination of the Ears

Weber Test

Hearing is tested with a 256 cycles per second (cps) or a 512-cps tuning fork. A 128-cps tuning fork measures vibration; it does not test hearing as well. The Weber test places the tuning fork in the center of the forehead and the physician asks the patient where he or she hears it (Fig. 1.1). Is it louder on one side than on the other or is it loudest in the center? With a normal Weber test, the sound is

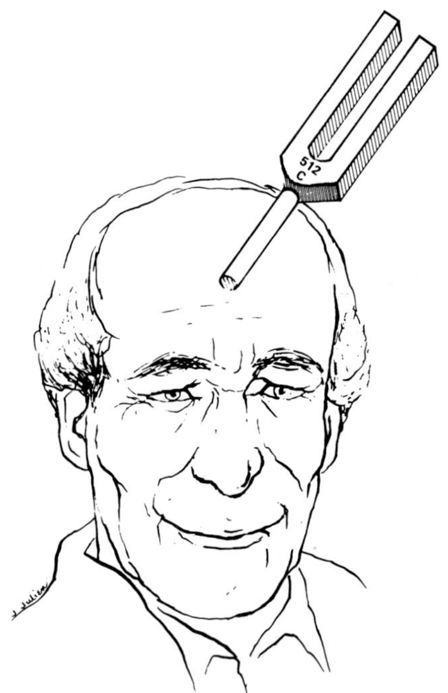

Figure 1.1. The Weber Test. A 256-cps or 512-cps tuning fork is placed on the forehead and the patient is asked, "Where do you hear that?" "Do you hear the noise in the center of your head or is it louder on one side or the other?" The patient may respond, "I hear it right up in front in the center of my forehead."

heard loudest in the center or it is heard equally in both ears. With an abnormal Weber test, the sound lateralizes, that is, it is heard louder in one ear. A lateralizing Weber test response is obvious to both patient and physician, but a midline Weber test response can be vague. The patient may not be certain exactly where he or she hears the sound, and it may be necessary to repeat the test several times. A Weber test will lateralize toward an ear with a middle ear conductive hearing loss. To understand this better, place a vibrating tuning fork on your own forehead. Move it to the right and to the left. Note how the sound also moves. Now create a conductive hearing loss by occluding your left external auditory canal with your finger. The sound now lateralizes to your left ear, no matter where on your forehead you place the tuning fork. With a sensorineural hearing loss—that is, one affecting the cochlea, the acoustic nerve, or, rarely, the brain— the Weber lateralizes away from the affected ear. If the sensorineural hearing loss is symmetrical as found with presbycusis, the hearing loss from aging, the Weber will be midline.

Rinne Test
Sound transmitted through an external ear traverses the middle ear and is perceived by the cochlea (inner ear). Sound can be transmitted directly to the cochlea, skipping the external and middle ear, by placing the vibrating tuning fork on the mastoid bone directly behind the ear. This is the basis for the Rinne hearing test. To perform this test, a 256-cps or 512-cps vibrating tuning fork is placed on the mastoid bone and then moved next to the external ear. The patient indicates at which of the two sites the sound is louder (Fig. 1.2). Normally, air conduction (AC) is greater than bone conduction (BC),

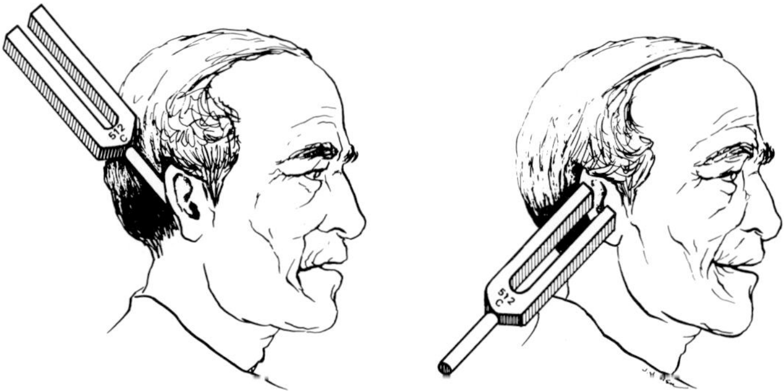

Figure 1.2. The Rinne Test. A 256-cps or 512-cps tuning fork is placed first on the mastoid bone (A) and then over the ear canal (B). The patient is asked, "Where is the sound louder: behind your ear or in your ear?" The patient should both hear and feel the vibration in A, and the sound should be louder in B.

a relationship written as Rinne AC > BC. If the bone conduction is greater, this implies that there is a conductive hearing deficit; that is, sound is not conducted through the external or the middle ear. Again, you can perform this test on yourself after creating a conductive hearing loss by occluding your left external auditory canal with your finger. Gross hearing can be tested by having the patient listen for the sound of two fingers rubbing together or whispering in the ear or, best, by having the patient affirm if he or she can hear the 256- or 512-cps tuning fork at a very low volume.

Audiometry

An audiogram is the best test for hearing. Air conduction is measured by placing earphones over both ears. Each ear is tested individually to determine its hearing threshold at 250, 500, 1000, 2000, 4000, 6000, and 8000 cps. Hearing is measured in decibels (dB), which is a logarithmic scale. Thresholds of hearing at 0 to 10 dB represent very good hearing; thresholds at 10 to 30 dB indicate a mild hearing loss; at 30 to 60 dB, there is a moderate hearing loss; at 60 to 90 dB, hearing loss is severe; and when the threshold is greater than 90 dB the individual is effectively deaf. By convention, air conduction thresholds for the right ear are indicated on the audiogram by the symbol "O" and for the left ear by an "X." Sensorineural hearing measures cochlear, eighth cranial nerve, brain stem, and cerebral auditory function. Sensorineural hearing is measured by placing a bone-conducting vibrator on the mastoid bone behind the ear. The same sound frequencies (250–8000 cps) are measured. Bone conduction on the right is indicated by the symbol "[" and on the left by the symbol "]." If air and bone conduction coincide, the air conduction is also a measure of sensorineural hearing and the bone conduction results are not recorded. Air conduction can never be better than bone conduction (sensorineural hearing). If air conduction is normal, it is not necessary to test bone conduction; only the air-conduction results are recorded.

Some patients have no trouble hearing pure tones, but still have difficulty hearing others talk. This is measured on the audiogram as speech reception threshold (SRT) and is recorded as a single number in decibels. The patient's ability to discriminate different words is also measured as discrimination ability and is recorded as a percentage. Discrimination percentages from 80% to 100% are considered good, 60% to 80% are acceptable, and less than 60% is poor. Figure 1.3 shows a normal audiogram.

Several variations and combinations of tuning fork and audiogram results can be found. Table 1.1 summarizes the Weber and the Rinne tuning fork tests found in clinical medicine. Tuning fork tests are not 100% reliable, but are a useful screening examination. They should correlate with the audiogram and if not, the tuning fork tests or the audiogram, or both, should be repeated until the results all appear

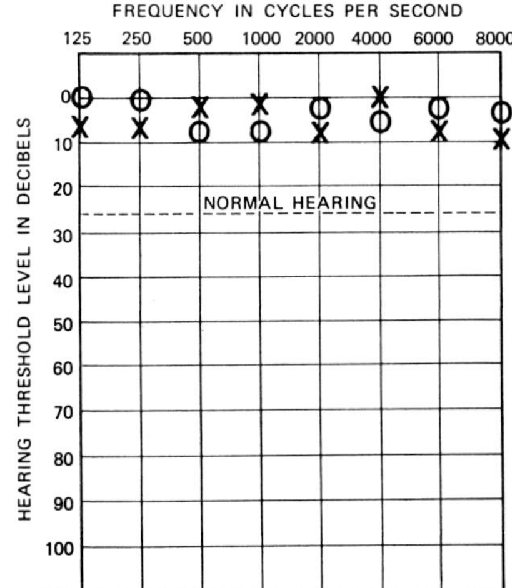

Figure 1.3. A standard audiogram report from a patient with normal hearing, good speech reception thresholds (SRT), and good word discrimination (Discrim). The sound levels are measured in decibels and recorded vertically. The different frequency sounds are recorded horizontally and measured in cycles per second (cps). The lower limits of normal hearing are indicated by the dashed line at about 25 dB.

Table 1.1 Tuning Fork Results

	WEBER*	RINNE*
Normal hearing	Midline	AC > BC AU
Conductive hearing loss		
Left	To the left	{ BC > AC AS AC > BC AD
Right	To the right	{ AC > BC AS BC > AC AD
Both	Midline	BC > AC AU
Sensorineural hearing loss		
Left	To the right	AC > BC AU
Right	To the left	AC > BC AU
Both	Midline	AC > BC AU

AC = air conduction, BC = bone conduction, AS = left ear, AD = right ear, AU = both ears.
*Tested with a 256- or 512-cps (cycle per second) tuning fork.

consistent. The following five cases illustrate some potential tuning fork and audiogram results.

A patient complains of decreased hearing in the left ear. The Weber test lateralizes to the left. Rinne test, BC > AC AS and AC > BC AD. (AS means auris sinister [left ear], AD means auris dexter [right ear], and AU means auris unitas [both ears].) The results suggest that the patient has a conductive hearing loss in the left ear (Fig. 1.4). The tuning fork tests and the audiogram demonstrate that this patient has a left ear conductive hearing loss. The SRT on the right is 5 dB, which is normal. On the left side the SRT is decreased to 20 dB, which is expected because of the left ear hearing loss. Discrimination in both ears, measured at 15 dB above the respective SRTs, is 96%, an excellent result.

Another patient complains of decreased hearing. Both ears seem equally involved. The Weber test is midline and bone conduction is greater than air conduction in both ears, suggesting a bilateral conductive hearing loss. The audiogram for this patient is shown in Figure 1.5.

The third patient complains of decreased hearing in the left ear. The Weber test lateralizes to the right ear. The Rinne test shows AC > BC AU. This suggests a left sensorineural hearing loss. The audiogram for this patient is shown in Figure 1.6. The tuning fork tests and the audiogram demonstrate that this patient has a left inner ear hearing loss (sensorineural hearing loss). The SRT in the right ear is 5 dB. The SRT in the left ear is decreased to 30 dB. Discrimination in the right ear is 96% when measured at 15 dB louder than the SRT. Discrimination on the left ear is decreased; it is 50% when measured at 15 dB louder than the SRT and is 65% when measured at 40 dB louder than the SRT.

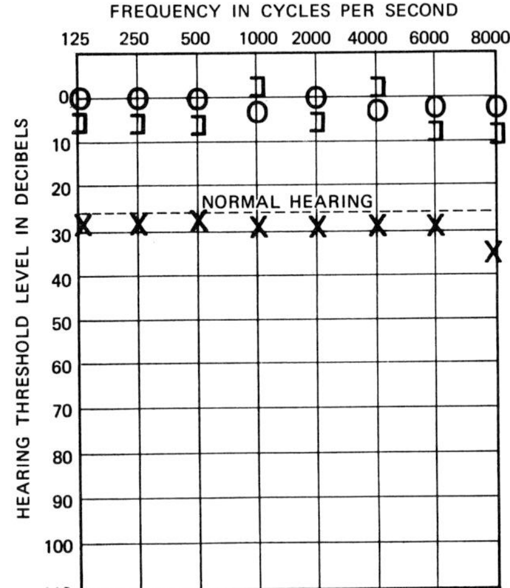

Figure 1.4. Audiogram of person with conductive hearing loss in the left ear. SRT = speech reception threshold; Discrim. = word discrimination.

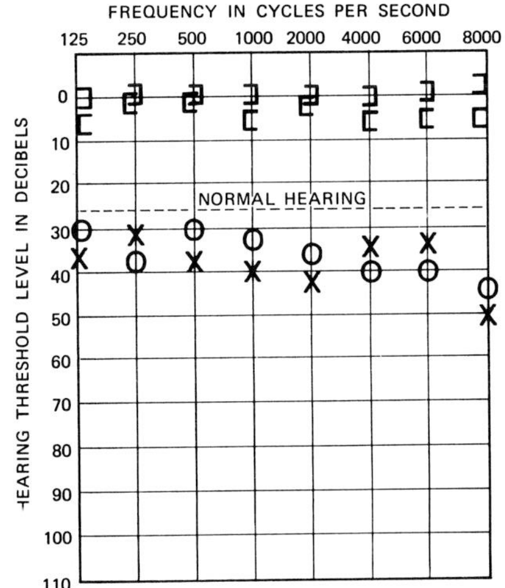

Figure 1.5. Audiogram of patient complaining of decreased hearing. SRT = speech reception threshold; Discrim. = word discrimination.

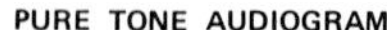

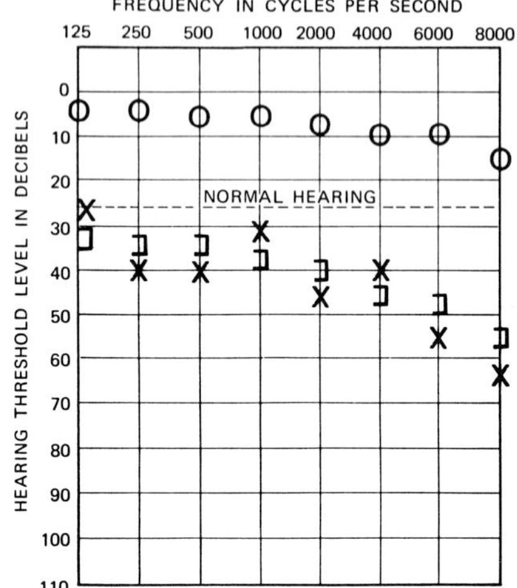

Figure 1.6. Audiogram of patient complaining of decreased hearing in left ear. SRT = speech reception threshold; Discrim. = word discrimination.

A fourth patient complains of decreased hearing in both ears. The Weber test is midline, and the Rinne test shows AC > BC AU. This suggests a bilateral sensorineural hearing loss. The audiogram for this patient is shown in Figure 1.7. The audiogram confirms the tuning fork tests. The SRTs are elevated in both ears, which is to be expected with this hearing loss. The discrimination is normal.

The last patient complains of decreased hearing in both ears. The Weber test is midline, and the Rinne test shows AC > BC AU. The audiogram reproduced in Figure 1.8 shows a moderate sensorineural hearing loss. Poor discrimination is noted. The patient hears pure tones satisfactorily, but cannot discriminate words. The ultimate effect is that the individual does not perceive language.

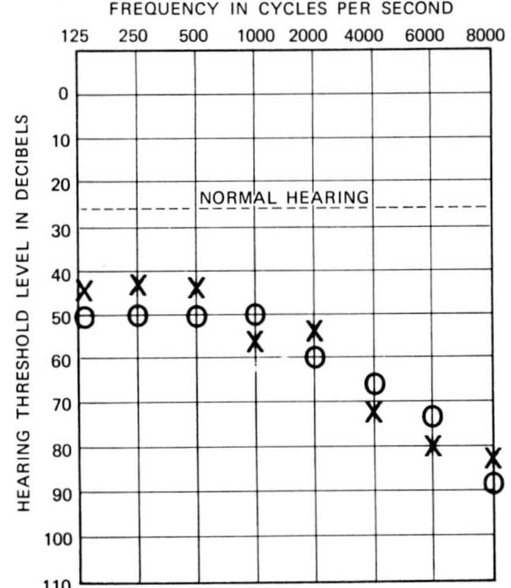

Figure 1.7. Audiogram of a patient with decreased hearing in both ears. SRT = speech reception threshold; Discrim. = word discrimination.

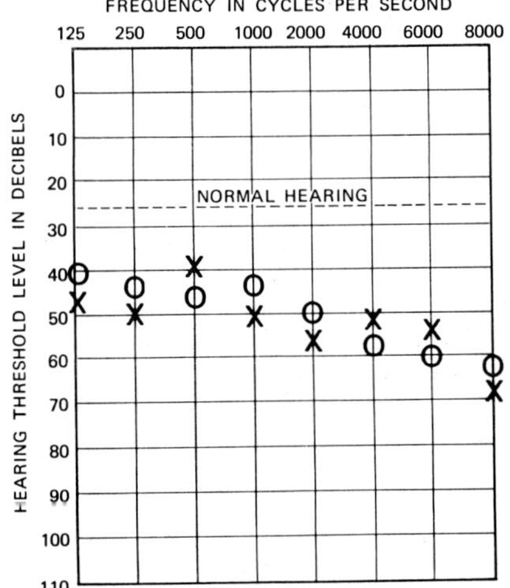

Figure 1.8. Audiogram of a patient with decreased hearing in both ears. SRT = speech reception threshold; Discrim. = word discrimination.

Other Tests of Hearing
When patients have mixed hearing losses—that is, conductive and sensorineural—tuning forks become very poor testers, and an audiogram will be necessary to determine the nature of these hearing losses. Additional tests are available to measure hearing functions.

Tympanometry measures the sound transmitted by the tympanic membrane at different middle ear pressures. It is useful for distinguishing different causes of conductive hearing losses and for measuring middle ear pressures. It also identifies the presence or absence of the stapedial reflex, which is a seventh cranial nerve function.

Brain stem-evoked-response audiometry (BERA) measures nerve potentials from the eighth cranial nerve and from the brain stem. It is useful for testing hearing in infants and for detecting cerebellopontine angle tumors.

Brain stem-evoked–response audiometry is rapidly gaining popularity as an important addition to the neurotologic evaluation. This method does not require patient participation, as does standard pure tone audiometry. It is extremely useful in localizing retrocochlear causes of sensorineural hearing loss. Figure 1.9 shows a normal tracing and correlates the different waves with their presumed respective anatomic origins. Both the wave forms and their respective latencies are important.

The *electronystagmogram* is useful in measuring vestibular function.

Anatomy of the Ear and Mechanism of Hearing
The anatomy of the ear should be known to all who deal with hearing disorders, but basic structures are reviewed here so that all will use the same terminology (see Fig. 1.10). The external ear canal is supported by cartilage laterally and by bone medially. Hairs and cerumen glands are present in the lateral third of the ear canal. The tympanic membrane, which lies at the medial end of this "sound tunnel," is very thin and supported about its circumference by a bony annulus. In this center, the tympanic membrane is attached firmly to the malleus. The middle ear is a small cavity connected with the nasopharynx through the eustachian tube. It is continuous, with the mastoid air cells behind the ear. The middle ear contains three small ear bones: the malleus, the incus, and the stapes. Sound transmitted through the external auditory canal causes the tympanic membrane to vibrate. This vibration is transmitted through and amplified 20 times by the middle ear (tympanic membrane, malleus, incus, and stapes). Sound enters the inner ear through the oval window. The sound is then perceived by the hair cells in the inner ear (cochlea) and is transmitted to the brain by the eighth cranial nerve. The round window is connected to the cochlea and is responsible for equalizing inner ear pressure. The vestibular system, containing the semicircular canals, is responsible for balance. It is intimately connected to the cochlea. The

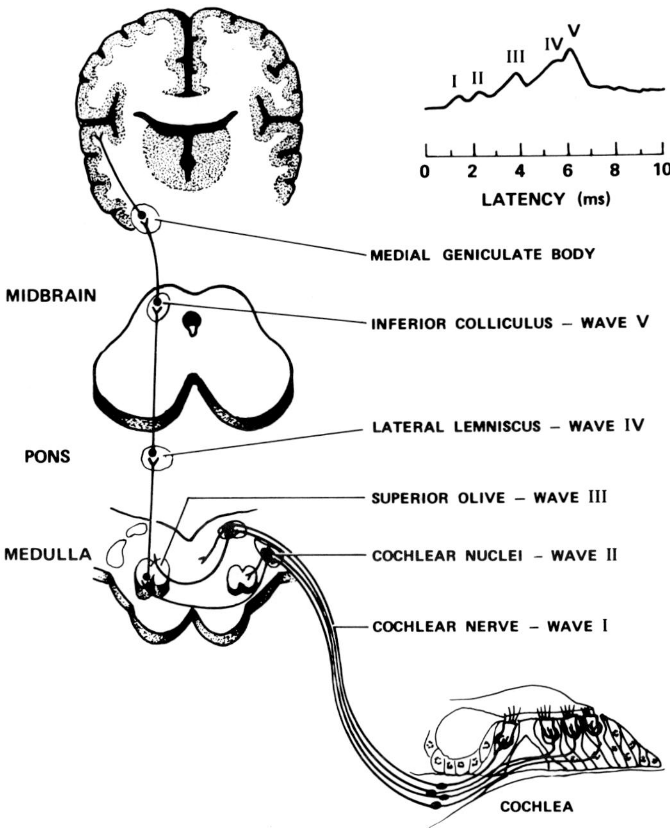

Figure 1.9. Anatomic correlation of audiometric brain stem-evoked-response potentials. (Used with permission of Dr. Jeffrey P. Harris.)

signals of the vestibular system to the brain are also carried by the eighth cranial nerve. The facial nerve runs through the inner ear, middle ear, and mastoid. The carotid artery, sigmoid sinus, and jugular bulb also course through the temporal bone.

Physical Examination of the Ear
Physical examination of the ear is difficult. The auricle and the lateral external ear canal are easily seen. The medial external ear canal and the tympanic membrane require an otoscope. The normal tympanic

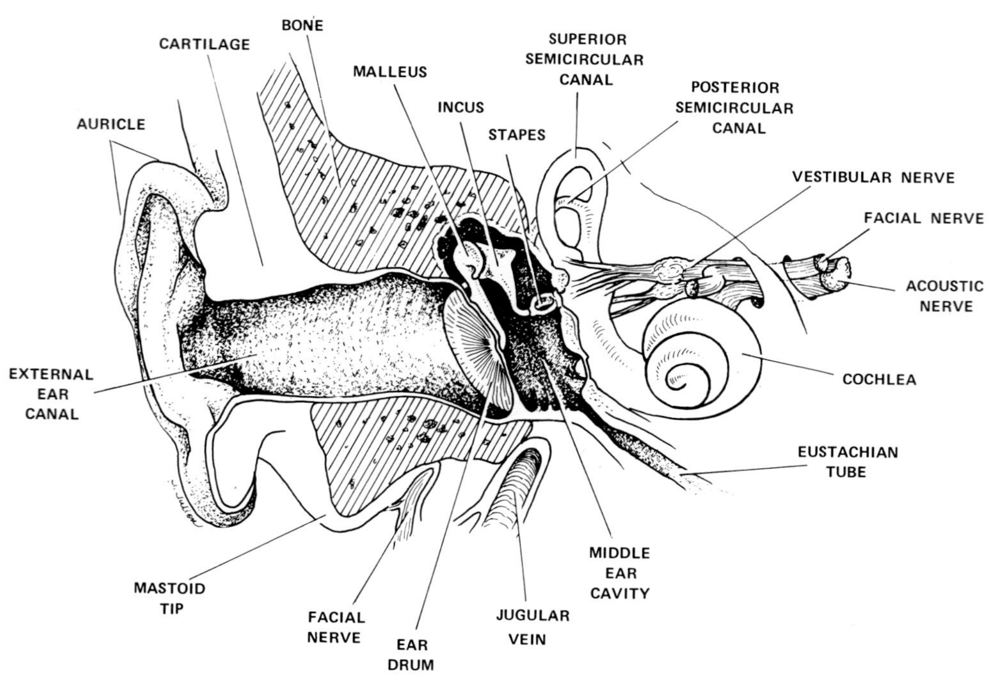

Figure 1.10. Anatomy of the ear.

membrane is translucent, gray in color, and may have vascular streaks along the malleus. If the throat is inflamed, as in otitis media, it thickens and loses its transparency. As it becomes increasingly inflamed, it becomes erythematous. The normal tympanic membrane lies in a neutral position. In otitis media, the middle ear contains a purulent exudate under pressure and this bulges the drum laterally. In serous otitis media, conversely, the middle ear has a decreased pressure and the drum is retracted medially. Drum position is difficult to determine with monocular vision. Incidentally, the presence of a light reflex has no meaning except to let you know you remembered to turn on the light on your otoscope.

Pneumomassage will help in evaluation of middle ear pressure. The otoscope speculum is placed so it gently seals the external ear canal. When the bulb on the otoscope is gently squeezed, the drum should visibly move away (medially) and then back (laterally). This is called normal movement to pneumomassage. If the drum is already retracted medially, it will not move when the bulb is squeezed. When the bulb

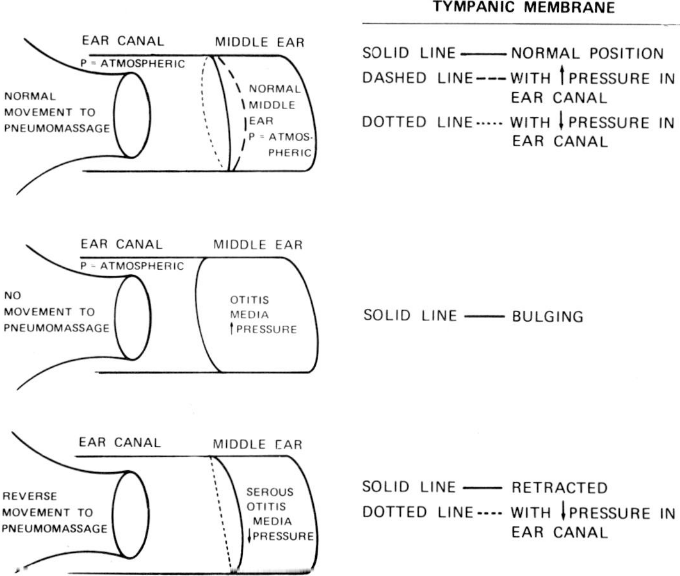

Figure 1.11. Pneumomassage. A great deal can be learned about the middle ear by applying pressure to the tympanic membrane, a procedure called pneumomassage. If it is done well, three different responses can be seen as depicted here. A severe negative pressure can pull the ear drum medially, and it too may exhibit no movement on pneumomassage.

is released, a negative pressure is created, and the drum will move laterally for an instant and then quickly back to its retracted position. This is called reverse movement to pneumomassage and is diagnostic of negative middle ear pressure. If the drum is under pressure and bulging laterally, it will not move at all to pneumomassage. Figure 1.11 illustrates these situations.

If a perforation is seen, its position and size should be noted. It is best to draw a picture of the drum and the perforation. It should be noted if the perforation extends to the margin or annulus of the drum (marginal perforation). Perforation that does not extend to the margin is called a central perforation. Figure 1.12 illustrates the most common perforations.

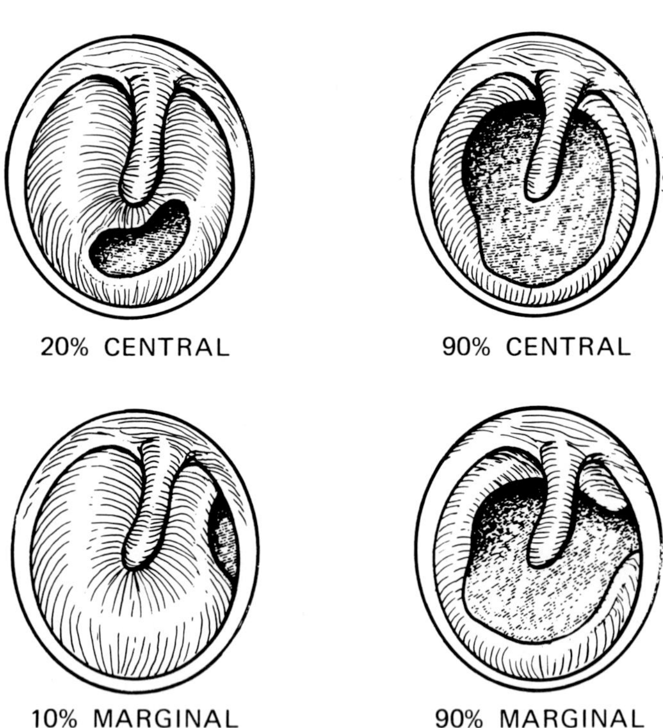

Figure 1.12.   Tympanic membrane perforations. If a tympanic membrane perforation is seen, you should draw a simple picture, estimate its size (in percentage), and indicate if it is marginal or central.

Examination of the Nose

If the external nose is deformed, it should be indicated, if not, it need not be mentioned. The interior of the nose should be examined either with a nasal speculum or otoscope speculum. If a speculum is used for the nose, it must be carefully washed with soap and water, alcohol, or other disinfectant between patients.

The septum and the middle and inferior turbinates should be visible. The mucosal color must be examined; inflammation turns the mucosa red. Allergy swells the mucosa and it appears pale or bluish in color. Polyps or tumors must be looked for deep in the nose. Today, the nasal cavity is better examined with a flexible or rigid endoscope. The flexible scopes are easier to use and provide a view of the larynx as well. Rigid endoscopes provide the best examination, but these are expensive and require topical nasal anesthesia. Rhinologists use the rigid endoscopes almost exclusively and can usually see all the turbinates, the entire nasal cavity, the major sinus ostia, and the nasopharynx.

Examination of the Throat (Oral Cavity, Oropharynx, Larynx, and Neck)

The nasopharynx can only be examined with special endoscopic instruments or a head light and a mirror. This normally is not part of a routine physical examination except when performed by a head and neck surgeon.

The oral cavity is examined by inspection and palpation and all the mucosal surfaces and the patient's teeth examined. The tonsils, the palate, and the pharynx must be observed, as well as palpate the palate, the cheeks, the tongue, the floor of the mouth, and the lips. If a pathologic condition exists in the posterior pharynx or nasopharynx, it is easily detected by palpation.

The larynx is examined with endoscopic instruments or with a mirror and head light. Most physicians do not examine the larynx routinely, but the techniques can be learned from any head and neck surgeon.

The neck is examined by palpating the pertinent structures in a routine systematic fashion. The posterior triangles are palpated while standing in front of the patient. The anterior triangles are palpated while standing behind the patient, beginning with the submental area. The submandibular gland can be located high under the mandible or can be ptotic, that is, hanging down lower in the neck. The hyoid, thyroid, and cricoid cartilages are palpated, followed by the internal jugular lymph node chain and finally the thyroid gland. The posterior cervical triangle is palpated, feeling for lymph nodes and abnormal masses. The area over the carotids is ausculated for bruits.

As stated at the start of this chapter, the examination is complex. Guidance and practice are needed to achieve competence.

CHAPTER 2

The Ear

The ear is a small, complex structure with several important functions. Disorders of the ear are common and may range in severity from minor complaints to incapacitating diseases. Many problems are easily recognized and treated; others are complex and require special knowledge and skill.

AURICULAR HEMATOMA

A typical history of an auricular hematoma is that of a high school wrestler who has been held in a rather fierce head lock, following which his ear has become swollen and painful. Examination reveals only a swollen ear with loss of the usual fine detail on the anterior lateral surface of the ear. The swelling is fluctuant and extremely painful to the touch. (Permission should be obtained to touch the ears and when received, should be done gently.)

The swelling is a hematoma located beneath the perichondrium and it lifts the perichondrium away from the cartilage. The entire blood supply to the cartilage comes from the perichondrium and loss of this blood supply will result in a severe fibrous reaction with consequent auricular deformity, which creates a rather thick, deformed, unattractive ear, known as a "cauliflower ear."

The hematoma must be drained. A 20-mL syringe and an 18-gauge needle are used. The ear should be swabbed gently with povidone-iodine and then alcohol. The needle is inserted and the blood clot aspirated. If this is successful, the patient should be observed for 30 minutes. If there is no reaccumulation of blood, it is important to advise the patient against taking aspirin or nonsteroidal anti-inflammatory drugs (NSAIDs) because they interfere with platelet aggregation and may predispose to further bleeding. Acetaminophen should be recommended. A mastoid dressing can be applied to maintain pressure, keeping skin coapted to the cartilage. The patient should return immediately if the swelling recurs. Wrestling or participation in any contact sport should not be allowed for 7 to 10 days.

If the blood clot cannot be aspirated, or if it recurs, it should be drained. After appropriate patient discussion and consent, the ear should be cleansed with povidone-iodine and the inferior extent of the hematoma injected with 1% xylocaine with 1:100,000 epinephrine. A 5-mm (stab) incision is made with a No. 11 knife blade, and the hematoma is removed with suction or massage. Some surgeons favor placing a small drain in the wound; others do not think a drain is necessary to permit new blood to escape. Also, a drain may serve as a tract for bacteria and cause a local infection. A pressure dressing, also called a mastoid dressing, must be applied. A dressing 36 inches iong (91.24 cm) of $\frac{1}{2}$-inch gauze is saturated with an antibiotic and petrolatum mixture, eg, povidone-iodine or bacitracin. The gauze should be placed against the ear, and packed in such a way that it will fill the depressions and concavities. It is necessary to pack it behind the ear as well, to support the ear away from the head. Several 4 × 4-inch gauze sponges can be placed over this, and the entire compress held on with 3-inch gauze wrapped around the head. The patient should be placed on oral cephalosporin prophylaxis for 48 hours. If the patient is in pain, a prescription for acetaminophen with 30 mg codeine is recommended. Again, the patient should be advised against taking aspirin or NSAIDs for any reason. The dressing should be changed after 12 to 24 hours, and removed after 3 days.

If infection or perichondritis is present at the time of presentation or develops during treatment, parenteral antibiotics should be given as directed by culture and sensitivity. The most common organisms are *Staphylococcus, Streptococcus pneumonia,* and occasionally *Pseudomonas aeruginosa.*

OTITIS EXTERNA (SWIMMER'S EAR)

Otitis externa is a common disease in individuals of all ages and both sexes. The patient may complain of pain, itching, or loss of hearing. In cases with acute onset, pain is predominant; in cases with slow onset, itching is predominant. There is usually a history of swimming, of playing in the water, or of trauma to the ear. The most common causes of otitis externa are cotton-tipped swabs.

P. aeruginosa is a normal inhabitant of the external ear. Its numbers are kept in balance by the normal acidity of the external auditory canal. Prolonged swimming or abusive use of cotton-tipped applicators alters the pH, producing a more basic environment, in which the *Pseudomonas* grows profusely. This causes a rapid epithelial desquamation, seen as a white debris filling the external auditory canal. An intensive inflammatory reaction occurs, and a perichondritis develops that causes the intense pain. This pain is easily elicited by grasping the auricle and shaking it gently—a sign that is pathognomonic for otitis externa. The ear canal is swollen and occasionally swells shut. The canal skin, if visible, is reddened.

Treatment

Treatment of *P. aeruginosa* infection is simple. If the patient is in the habit of inserting cotton-tipped applicators, bobby pins, or other objects into the ear, the practice should be stopped. If the ear is filled with a white, desquamated epithelium, it should be gently suctioned clean. The mainstay of treatment is ear drops. Many brands of commercial ear drops are available. They all contain an acidifying agent and a drying agent—two important ingredients. Most also contain a combination of antibiotics and steroids; most physicians use these combination ear drops. Cortisporin otic is popular. The solution is preferable to the suspension because it permits better subsequent inspection. Prescribe a 10-cc bottle; 2 to 3 drops in the affected ear three to four times daily. Symptoms usually disappear within 1 to 2 days. If the patient cannot afford to purchase a commercial product, a home remedy can be made by mixing equal volumes of vinegar, 70% isopropyl alcohol, and tap water. This solution works well but is slightly odoriferous.

If the ear canal is swollen shut, a small cotton wick 2-mm wide and 10-mm long can be made by twisting cotton around a metal applicator. This can then be inserted into the outer one half of the ear canal. The wick is removed after 3 to 4 days. There is no need for oral antibiotics. Otitis external is a painful malady and often requires aspirin with 30 mg codeine every 3 to 4 hours. Heat from a heating pad or hot water bottle is also effective.

Occasionally, a patient, most often a diabetic, does not respond to local therapy and experiences intense pain. The condition may be osteomyelitis of the temporal bone, also called malignant otitis externa, which has a high mortality rate. The patient should be referred to a head and neck surgeon and hospitalized immediately.

EXTERNAL AUDITORY CANAL EXOSTOSES (SURFER'S EAR)

This is an increasingly common and fascinating problem found in patients with a long history of cold-water exposure. It is found almost exclusively in surfers and professional divers. Often, the patient will present with otitis externa. On examination, a sprinkling of beach sand and two or three large, white, hard growths are seen in the medial third of the external ear canal. If these growths are large, they will obstruct the view of the tympanic membrane. If they occlude more than 50% of the ear canal lumen, they can cause recurrent otitis externa. Particularly if the patient plans to continue exposure to cold water, the exostoses should be removed. This difficult operation should be performed by an otologist.

OTITIS MEDIA—MIDDLE EAR INFECTIONS

Otitis media is divided into three categories: acute, serous, and chronic.

Acute Otitis Media

Almost all children have at least one bout of acute otitis media before the age of 5 years. Otitis media is the second most common reason for children to see a pediatrician. A typical history is that of a preschool child developing an upper respiratory viral infection that ultimately becomes a purulent rhinorrhea (runny nose). Just about the time the parents think they are finished with a drippy nose, the child becomes cranky and febrile. At 1 year of age, children bat or tug at the affected ear, and by 2 or 3 years, they complain of pain. Adults with otitis media complain of pain (often intense), a pressure or a feeling of fullness, and a hearing loss. Examination shows the classic red, bulging tympanic membrane of otitis media. The Weber test lateralizes to the infected ear, and the Rinne test reveals BC > AC, that is, there is a conductive hearing loss.

The organisms involved in acute otitis media are the upper respiratory tract bacteria described in Box 2.1. In patients without bacterial infections, viruses may be found. The pathogenesis is different among individuals. Normally, the eustachian tube allows air into the middle ear space and is a conduit to drain the mucous secretions of the mastoid and middle ear. A normally functioning eustachian tube should prevent reflux of secretions from the nasopharynx. When the eustachian tube is not functioning properly, the middle ear is not aerated, middle ear and mastoid secretions do not drain, and there may be reflux of nasopharyngeal fluids and bacteria.

Box 2.1. Bacteriology of Otitis Media

Acute suppurative otitis media is usually attributed to the *Streptococcus pneumoniae* or *Hemophilus influenzae* organisms. Most surveys rate pneumococcal infections as more common; others note an equal or higher incidence of hemophilus, which causes infections not only in children, but also in adolescents and occasionally in adults. During the past 50 years there has been a steady increase in the proportion of hemophilus infections coincident with a progressive decline in streptococcal otitis media (*Streptococcus pyogenes*, beta-hemolytic group A). More recently, a significant increase has been seen in the prevalence of *Moraxella (AKA Branhamella,* and before that *Neisseria) catarrhalis,* which is pathogenic. Ampicillin resistance by hemophilus runs about 20 percent nationwide and by *B. catarrhalis* up to 75 percent. *Staphylococcus aureus* is unusual enough that it need not be considered in initial therapy. Many studies show about 25 to 30 percent no growth from middle ear aspirate cultures. This group is smaller if techniques are used to culture fastidious organisms such as *Mycoplasma pneumoniae*, anaerobic bacteria, and other low virulence bacteria such as *Staphylococcus epidermidis* and diphtheroids, the significance of which is not known. Viruses (eg, respiratory synctial) can be isolated also.

Acute mastoiditis (in the absence of chronic suppurative otitis media) is most likely caused by *S. pneumoniae*, but *S. pyogenes* and *S. aureus* are almost as frequent pathogens. Recently, anaerobic organisms (ie, *Bacteroides fragilis* and *melanogenicus*) have also been implicated. Mastoiditis is rarely due to *H. influenzae*, which causes mucus membrane infections but may be less invasive to bone. *M. tuberculosis* is occasionally encountered, particularly in immigrants from third world nations.

Bullous myringitis has been noted as an accompanying complaint in experimental studies of acute pulmonary infections in young adults. The *M. pneumoniae* organism was implicated, but its role in isolated tympanic membrane infection is not so clear. In children the same organisms of acute otitis media are found in bullous myringitis.

S. pneumoniae	25%
H. influenzae	20–25%
B. catarrhalis	10–20%
S. pyogenes (gr. A)	2%
S. aureus	1%
Others	20%
Mixed infections	5%
No growth	Remainder

Modified from Stool and Bluestone. Antimicrobial Therapy in Otolaryngology-Head and Neck Surgery, 5th edition, Fairbanks, D.N.F., with permission.

A number of eustachian tube dysfunctions can cause or predispose to infection of the middle ear. For example, infected secretions may reflux from the diseased nasopharynx. Alternatively, the eustachian tube may be obstructed because of inflammation from infection or allergy. Large adenoids or a nasopharyngeal neoplasm will obstruct the eustachian tube. Air no longer enters the middle ear and fluids no longer drain. A perfect culture medium is set up: bacteria from the nasopharynx invade, and otitis media begins.

The mastoid is a system of air cells intimately connected with the middle ear. The mastoid air cells drain through the middle ear and the eustachian tube and into the nasopharynx. Both the mastoid and the middle ear are lined with upper respiratory tract mucosa. When the middle ear is infected, the mastoid cells also are infected. Therefore, all patients with acute otitis media also have acute mastoiditis. This condition is discussed more fully later in this chapter.

Treatment

Treatment for acute otitis medias in adults consists of 250 mg to 500 mg oral amoxicillin three times daily for 10 days. Infections in children under the age of 5 years have a significant incidence of colonization with penicillin-resistant *Hemophilus influenzae* and are best treated with amoxicillin 40 mg/kg/d (maximum 1 g/d), divided into three daily doses and given for 10 days. Patients allergic to penicillins are treated with appropriate doses of erythromycin. One brand of sulfamethoxazole, Septra®, has gained popularity among some physicians because it tastes good and is given only twice daily, but it is not yet the drug of choice. It should be saved for resistant otitis media or for children who absolutely will not take amoxicillin. An alternative drug therapy is penicillin and sulfonamide, but this too is saved for patients who do not respond to amoxicillin. The antibiotics used in otitis media therapy are shown in Table 2.1.

Occasionally, children develop four or more episodes of recurrent otitis media yearly. They may do well with prophylactic therapy; once-daily amoxicillin or twice-daily sulfisoxazole are most commonly used. A child who develops acute otitis media with every occurrence of upper respiratory tract infection (RTI) is best treated

**Table 2.1 Concentration of Antibiotics Used in Children
with Acute Otitis Media**

DRUG	DOSAGE (mg/kg)
1st Line	
Ampicillin	80 mg/kg/24 h in 4 doses
Amoxicillin	40 mg/kg/24 h in 3 doses
2nd Line	
Cefaclor	40 mg/kg/24 h in 3 doses
Erythromycin and sulfisoxasole	40 mg (.067 cc) erythromycin/kg/24 h in 4 doses
Trimethoprim and sulfamethoxazole	8 mg trimethoprim and 40 mg sulfamethoxazole in 2 doses
3rd Line	
Amoxicillin & clavulanic acid	40 mg/kg/24 h in 3 doses
Cefixime	8 mg/kg/24 h in 1 or 2 doses

prophylactically with 10 days of amoxicillin therapy every time a runny nose develops. Nose drops, decongestants, antihistamines, herbs, and even Carter's Little Liver Pills have been given as well, but only the antibiotics have proved effective. The patient should have a follow-up visit at 10 to 14 days to ensure that the ear infection has cleared, and this should be continued at 2-week intervals until the ear is completely normal.

Occasionally in an acute infection, the tympanic membrane perforates. Green or yellow pus is then present in the external auditory canal. Culture of the pus is rarely of therapeutic significance and thus is not necessary, however, the infection should be treated with antibiotic ear drops such as Cortisporin Otic Solution® (Burroughs Wellcome) and appropriate oral antibiotics prescribed.

Neonatal Otitis Media
If a neonate (less than 6 weeks old) develops otitis media, there is a significant risk that *Escherichia coli, Bacteroides,* or other gram-negative bacteria are responsible. Tympanocentesis is recommended for diagnosis and culture before beginning antibiotic therapy. This procedure, usually performed by a head and neck surgeon, involves aspirating the middle ear contents with a 22- or 25-gauge needle under the microscope. The child can be immobilized for this, and no anesthesia is used. The aspirate is Gram stained, a culture obtained, and sensitivity tests performed. If enteric organisms, presumably acquired during exit from the birth canal, are found, the child is admitted to the hospital and treated with appropriate intravenous (IV) antibiotics. If the infant is less than 4 weeks old, there is significant risk that his or her immune system may not be able to contain the otitis media. Therefore, all children less than 4 weeks of age are hospitalized, treated with IV antibiotics, and observed carefully for sepsis. An infant older than 4 weeks with a gram-negative infection should be admitted to the hospital and treated with IV antibiotics. If the child is more than 8 weeks old and is found to have the usual gram-positive upper respiratory tract organisms, he or she can be treated as an outpatient with amoxicillin 40 mg/kg/d given in three equal doses. Some infants between 4 and 8 weeks of age with gram-positive organisms are admitted to the hospital for IV antibiotics and observation for sepsis, whereas others can be treated adequately with oral antibiotics and observation at home.

Mastoiditis
The acute mastoiditis associated with acute otitis media generally resolves as the middle ear infection resolves. Occasionally, the mastoid does not drain normally through the middle ear and, in fact, becomes an abscess in and of itself, a condition called coalescent mastoiditis. It occurs most commonly in a patient who has had acute otitis media that has been incompletely treated with antibiotics. The

symptoms from the otitis media resolve, but approximately 2 to 3 weeks later the patient becomes acutely ill. The middle ear may or may not appear normal. Typically, a tenderness and swelling is evident behind the ear, and in severe cases, the ear may even protrude out away from the head. An X ray will confirm an inflammatory process in the mastoid air cells. Frequently, many of the small septa within the mastoid are destroyed. Because this is an abscess, it requires drainage—a surgical procedure called mastoidectomy.

Case Studies: Neonatal Otitis Media

Two case examples will illustrate the uniqueness of neonatal otitis media. The first is a 1-week-old baby boy of normal gestation and delivery. The infant went home 3 days after delivery and was well until the morning of the seventh day, when he became somewhat irritable, stopped feeding, and vomited more than was normal. The parents brought him to an emergency department. The infant appeared relatively well and had sustained his birth weight. On physical examination, the physician was unable to visualize the eardrums well, believed that the throat and neck examination findings were normal, the lungs clear, and the abdomen soft with good bowel sounds. A urine specific was clear, with no evidence of bacteria or white cells. The doctor was uneasy about his inability to see the eardrum and so made a presumptive diagnosis of otitis media and placed the child on oral amoxicillin and sent him home. The infant did not feed that evening but the next morning seemed to be a little better. Again the next evening, he had some difficulty with feeding and regurgitated. The child did not wake in the middle of the night and the parents, who were exhausted from the events of the previous 2 days, did not themselves waken. When they went to check on the child in the morning, he was dead.

An autopsy was performed and it was found that the infant had died of septic shock. *Escherichia coli* was cultured from his blood, his heart, and his kidney. Because of the diagnosis of otitis media, a head and neck surgeon was asked to examine the ears. A myringotomy was performed and the middle ear was found to be filled with pus, from which *E. coli* was cultured. The final diagnosis was otitis media caused by *E. coli,* and the cause of death was disseminated *E. coli* infection and septic shock.

The second patient was a 6-week-old baby boy, also normal gestation and delivery. At 6 weeks of age, the child became somewhat listless, did not feed as well as usual, and also vomited a few times, which was uncommon for this baby. The parents brought him to the emergency department; physical examination revealed a baby who had put on weight since birth and seemed to be quite healthy. The ears were difficult to examine, but the throat, neck, lungs, and abdomen were normal. The urine showed no evidence of bacteria or white cells. The doctor requested a head and neck surgery consultation because of his inability to see inside the ears. The head and neck surgeon also had difficulty visualizing the tympanic membrane with an otoscope, but using a microscope was able to see the eardrum, which appeared to be inflamed and thickened. A fine needle was inserted through the eardrum and the contents of the middle ear aspirated. This was sent to the laboratory for Gram staining and culture and sensitivity tests. The results showed gram-positive cocci in chains, and the diagnosis of a gram-positive coccal otitis media was made. There was then discussion about whether or not to admit the infant to the hospital for IV antibiotic therapy or permit him to be treated at home. Because the child was doing well and was now 6 weeks old and had a gram-positive coccal infection, it was elected to treat the child at home on oral amoxicillin. The child did well on this treatment plan. Had he been younger than 6 weeks or had gram-negative organisms been found, the infant ideally would have been admitted to the hospital for treatment.

The first child was incompletely evaluated, his condition was misdiagnosed, and he was mistreated. The second child was correctly evaluated, diagnosed, and treated.

Case Studies: Mastoiditis

A 9-year-old in San Diego developed pain in the ear and a markedly elevated temperature following an upper respiratory tract infection. She was seen in a free clinic. The diagnosis of acute otitis media was made, and she was given a prescription for ampicillin, which she took for the first 3 days but then developed diarrhea and discontinued. By this time, her fever was gone and the diarrhea stopped shortly after stopping the ampicillin. The child did well for the next week and a half, but then again began developing fever and pain, this time behind the ear. Her parents put her back on the ampicillin. Three days later, she was brought to the hospital comatose. Examination of the ear showed a gray, thickened tympanic membrane. There was a soft, spongy inflammation behind the ear. A myringotomy was performed, and pus was aspirated from the middle ear. A middle ear ventilation tube was placed. A Gram stain was suggestive of *Hemophilus influenzae*. A lumbar puncture was performed, and the cerebrospinal fluid was found to be loaded with white cells and bacteria. After much discussion, it was decided that this patient had meningitis secondary to an inadequately treated otitis media. The otitis media had developed into a coalescent mastoiditis, and the infection in the mastoid had spread to the cerebrospinal fluid, either in the middle fossa or in the posterior fossa, both of which lie immediately adjacent to the mastoid. A mastoidectomy was performed. Indeed, there was a coalescent mastoiditis with erosion of bone and a direct communication into the middle fossa. The child was then treated with IV antibiotics and regained consciousness shortly after surgery. Unfortunately, as a result of the meningitis there was a tremendous inflammatory reaction around the eighth cranial nerve at its entrance to the internal auditory canal, and this child developed a profound sensorineural hearing loss in both ears.

A second case example illustrates another common problem with ear disease. It is more frequently seen in Mexicans and in Eskimos, but occurs in other groups as well. The patient was a 9-year-old when he developed an acute otitis media. Medical services were not available to him. On the third day of his infection the eardrum ruptured, the pain immediately ceased, and defervescence occurred. After 3 days of purulent otorrhea, the patient was well. Over the next 10 years, he would occasionally develop a recurrent ear infection that always resulted in a purulent drainage from the affected ear. At the age of 20 years, he sought medical attention because of a persistent foul smell emanating from the involved ear. Examination revealed a large posterior marginal perforation with cholesteatomatous debris clearly evident. Mastoid X rays showed a poorly pneumatized mastoid on the involved side with evidence of a cholesteatoma eroding into the mastoid. A tympanomastoidectomy was performed. The cholesteatoma had eroded most of the incus and all of the suprastructure of the stapes. It was also eroding into the mastoid. The facial nerve was dehiscent where it lay adjacent to the cholesteatoma. All of the cholesteatoma was removed and a tympanoplasty was performed. This man healed well. Six months later, the middle ear was explored. There was no evidence of recurrent cholesteatoma, and the ossicles were reconstructed. The patient healed well after this operation and had good improvement in hearing.

Serous Otitis Media (Otitis Media with Effusion)

Poor eustachian tube function is particularly common in small children (aged 1 to 3 years) who do not yet have eustachian tubes long enough or oriented at the correct angle to protect their middle ears. Antimicrobial therapy commonly will sterilize the middle ear but leave a persistent serous exudate called serous otitis media. The condition can also occur in children and adults de novo, that is not preceded by acute otitis media. Serous otitis media is recognized by otoscopy. The tympanic membrane is a gray or amber color, may have air bubbles or an air–fluid level behind it, and, because of the negative pressure is retracted and draped about the middle ear ossicles. Pneumomassage will reveal a drum that either does not move at all or has reverse movement. Older patients complain of hearing loss. Tympanometry reveals a negative pressure, and tuning forks and audiometry indicate a conductive hearing loss. The diagnosis is usually made clinically. Audiologic testing is ordered only for difficult cases or to document the degree of hearing loss in patients with chronic cases.

To treat serous otitis media properly, the cause should be understood and treated. Poor eustachian tube function is more common in children, but is also found in adults. Eustachian tube dysfunction is a term used when no other diagnosis can be made.

Many conditions may precede serous otitis media. Upper respiratory tract allergy often manifests as a chronic stuffy, runny nose. The same allergic process affects the eustachian tube and the middle ear. Allergy treatment with antihistamine decongestants or allergy testing and desensitization are indicated. Thick residual fluid from otitis media is another common prelude to serous otitis media. Examination looks for nasopharyngeal obstruction. The adenoids are often causative in children. Tumors can cause obstruction in older children and adults. Angiofibroma is the most common nasopharyngeal tumor in pubertal males. Nasal polyps can obstruct the nasopharynx at any age. An older male or female patient must be examined for a nasopharyngeal carcinoma; unilateral serous otitis media in an adult should be considered cancer until proved otherwise. All children with cleft palates have poor eustachian tube function because of their palatal defect. Barotrauma sustained while flying or diving can also cause serous otitis media.

The nasopharynx should be examined with a mirror, looking up from the back of the oral cavity. This requires some physician skill in adults and is almost impossible with children. In adults and cooperative children, endoscopic examination of the nasopharynx may be performed through the nose (see Chapter 1). The nasopharynx can be seen on soft tissue lateral X rays, computed tomography (CT) scans, or xeroradiographs and are useful to evaluate adenoids in children. The CT scan is used to evaluate tumors in children and adults.

Finally, if needed to rule out tumor, the nasopharynx can be examined well under general anesthesia. This is most often done when there is suspicion of a tumor and a biopsy will be needed.

In adults, the nasopharynx is best examined endoscopically. As discussed in Chapter 1, flexible and rigid endoscopes can be used.

Treatment

Treatment for serous otitis media combines scientific rationale and empiric therapy. Identified predisposing causes are treated directly (allergies, upper respiratory tract infection (RTI), and so forth). Otherwise, the following therapeutic regimen is recommended. Simple observation for 2 weeks will often result in spontaneous resolution of effusion. If effusion persists, a decongestant is prescribed. Sudafed®, Entex®, and Naldecon® are common examples. Antihistamines are useful with an allergic rhinitis. Antihistamines tend to thicken secretions and may impede drainage of the effusion via the eustachian tube. If after 2 weeks of decongestant use the effusion persists, oral antibiotics (amoxicillin) in a dose appropriate to weight is added for 10 days. The rationale for antibiotic treatment is the presence of bacteria in about 30% of cultured, clinically noninfected effusions.

If the effusion persists, the antibiotic is changed and the decongestant continued. Occasionally, three different antibiotics may be necessary to clear an effusion. If effusion persists after three courses of antibiotics, myringotomy usually is indicated. At this point, specialty consultation with a head and neck surgeon is prudent. The specialist may try other medicines, simply observe the patient for 3 to 6 months, or, if the drum is severely retracted or a significant conductive hearing loss exists, recommend myringotomy and middle ear ventilation tubes. Normally, this can be done under local anesthesia in adults or with a mask general anesthesia in children 7 to 10 years. Using a binocular microscope, a small incision is made in the anterior inferior quadrant of the tympanic membrane and a small flanged Silastic tube is inserted (Fig. 2.1). This allows fluids to drain and air to enter. Normally the tube is extruded within a year, but if not, it can be removed easily. Patients, including young children, may swim and bathe with custom-fitted ear molds. Perforations requiring surgical closure occur in about 1% of patients.

If the surgeon believes the adenoids or tonsils, or both, play a significant role in a patient's disease, they can be removed at the same time as myringotomy. However, performing these procedures raises the morbidity and mortality rates and the cost of the surgery.

Chronic Otitis Media

Chronic otitis media is a far more serious disease than the other otitis medias. It is caused by perforation during an acute bout of otitis media (see Fig. 1.12 for types of perforations) or as a result of long-term

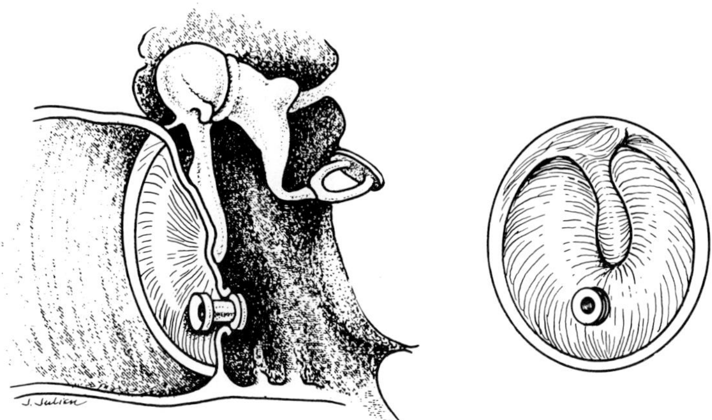

Figure 2.1. Middle ear ventilation tubes, called M&T's or PE tubes, are placed through the tympanic membrane and act as an artificial eustachian tube.

serous otitis media with severe retraction of the tympanic membrane. Some perforations, whether large or small, do not extend to the outer rim of the tympanic membrane (called the annulus); these are called central perforations. They often heal spontaneously, but if they do not, they are easily closed surgically. Sometimes the perforation extends to the annulus. This is dangerous, because now external auditory canal epithelium can grow down into the middle ear, ultimately forming a narrow-mouthed sac extending posteriorly and superiorly into the mastoid cavity. This development is called an epidermal inclusion cyst or cholesteatoma. Such a cyst is dangerous simply because of its location. Within 1 cm lie the cochlea, the vestibular labyrinth and semicircular canals, the carotid artery, the facial nerve, the sigmoid sinus, the jugular bulb, the middle cranial fossa, and the posterior cranial fossa. The inflammatory response within an epidermal inclusion cyst pushes it to expand, even erode, into bone. When it erodes into surrounding structures, severe complications can occur, including meningitis, brain abscess, total hearing loss, facial nerve paralysis, carotid artery blowout, or sigmoid sinus thrombosis with a resultant hydrocephalus.

Green or yellow pus is often present in the auditory canal in chronic otitis media. The foul smelling drainage is almost pathognomonic for the condition. A cholesteatoma necessitates mastoidectomy to eradicate the infection, to restore normal hearing, and to graft a new eardrum. The operation is performed from an incision behind the ear.

The mastoid bone is carefully drilled away under the microscope. The cholesteatoma is removed, and the normal anatomy is reconstructed. Depending on the extent of the disease and on the state of the eustachian tube, complete closure of the air-bone gap can sometimes be achieved, whereas at other times there is no improvement in hearing.

OTOSCLEROSIS

Otosclerosis is a fascinating familial disease that begins in the late teens, the 20s, or the 30s. It affects both men and women. In the latter, it tends to become evident during pregnancy. A typical history is that of a woman in her 20s who develops a unilateral ringing (tinnitus) during pregnancy. The tinnitus remains after delivery. She then notes a hearing loss in that ear. Typically, her mother had a similar experience, which ultimately may have affected both ears and made her almost completely deaf later in life. The patient does not have dizziness or take medications. Examination is normal, except that the Weber test lateralizes to the involved ear, and bone conduction is greater than air conduction Rinne test (BC > AC) with the 256-cps and 512-cps tuning forks. The tympanic membrane is normal. Audiometry confirms a conductive hearing loss.

The patient usually elects to have surgery, which involves lifting the tympanic membrane and examining the middle ear ossicles. The malleus and incus are normal, but the stapes is "fixed." The footplate of the stapes has developed exuberant bone growth and is fixed to the oval window by this growth. The stapes is removed (stapedectomy), and a prosthesis is fashioned to replace it. An older prosthesis is a small piece of fat taken from the ear lobe and tied to the end of a 4-mm long, thin piece of wire. A hook is fashioned at the other end and this is crimped to the incus. The eardrum is replaced, and the ear heals well. In 90% to 95% of cases, the ringing disappears and the patient's hearing returns to normal.

New techniques involve drilling a 0.6- to 0.8-mm hole in the stapedial footplate. This can be done by hand, by electric drill, or by laser. A teflon piston is inserted through the hole in the stapedial footplate. The other end is a wire crimped to the long process of the incus. With the newer technique, results are allegedly better and complications even less common. Possible complications of stapedectomy include total hearing loss, failure to improve hearing, persistent tinnitus, and temporary or permanent dizziness.

Most otosclerosis involves the stapes and oval window. Sometimes the cochlea is also involved, producing a sensorineural hearing loss. When cochlear otosclerosis occurs alone, a pure sensorineural hearing loss exists. Most commonly, cochlear otosclerosis is found with stapedial involvement; in these cases, a mixed (combined conductive and sensorineural) hearing loss will be present. The treatment for cochlear otosclerosis is controversial. Patients should be referred to a head and neck surgeon for treatment.

MENIERE'S DISEASE

Meniere's disease is relatively uncommon, but unfortunately this term has become a catch-all phrase for many disorders with symptoms of dizziness. It is an unpredictable, episodic disease. Patients have attacks of sudden hearing loss associated with tinnitus. They are vertiginous (dizzy) and describe a feeling of fullness in the ear. Other than the hearing loss, which is sensorineural, the entire neurotologic examination may be normal. The episodes are usually short in duration (hours to days) with gradual resolution of symptoms over weeks. A complete work-up for vertigo, as outlined later, can yield negative results. Etiology of the disease is unknown. Certain treatable causes of similar symptoms exist (syphilis, acoustic neuroma, perilymph fistula). In such cases, treatment directed toward the cause will relieve the vertigo. For idiopathic cases, phenothiazines, as outlined in the section on vertigo, are usually effective. A low-salt diet and daily use of diuretics is often helpful. Diazepam may also be effective. If none of these regimens is uniformly successful, the only recourse is to treat each attack symptomatically. If the disease progresses, as it frequently does, the patient develops an increasingly severe sensorineural hearing loss with each ensuing attack, even to the point of deafness. Permanent dizziness can occur. The vertigo and the tinnitus can be treated surgically, and patients with advanced cases should be considered for surgical therapy. The diagnosis of Meniere's disease should never be made until a work-up for vertigo is completed and until the disease is clearly shown to be episodic in nature. All new patients should have a complete vertigo work-up (see page 47) to exclude other causes of dizziness.

PRESBYCUSIS

Presbycusis is a type of hearing loss often found in aging patients. However, it can occur in people in their 30s. Histologically, there are hair-cell losses in the cochlea. Clinically, hearing decreases, initially in the high frequencies, but as the disease progresses, low frequencies are also affected. Speech discrimination deteriorates, and soon patients find they must ask people to repeat what they have said. Patients have the most difficulty trying to hear things against background-competing noises, such as music and party conversations. They also experience the phenomenon of recruitment, which causes them to hear loud noises as being unpleasantly loud. For example, when trying to listen to television or to a conversation, the patient has trouble hearing and so turns up the volume or asks friends to speak louder. When the noise reaches a certain level, it is suddenly too loud. Evaluation of hearing loss should include a history to determine whether the loss is of slow onset and to discover whether there has been intense noise exposure. When presbycusis is present, the otologic examination will be normal. Audiograms will show a typical pattern (Figs. 2.2 and 2.3). Sometimes speech discrimination

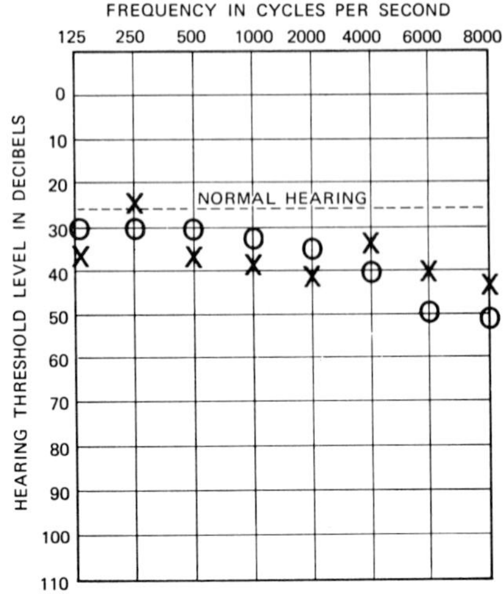

Figure 2.2. Typical audiogram of a patient with mild sensorineural hearing loss. Diagnosis: presbycusis. SRT = speech reception threshold; Discrim = word discrimination.

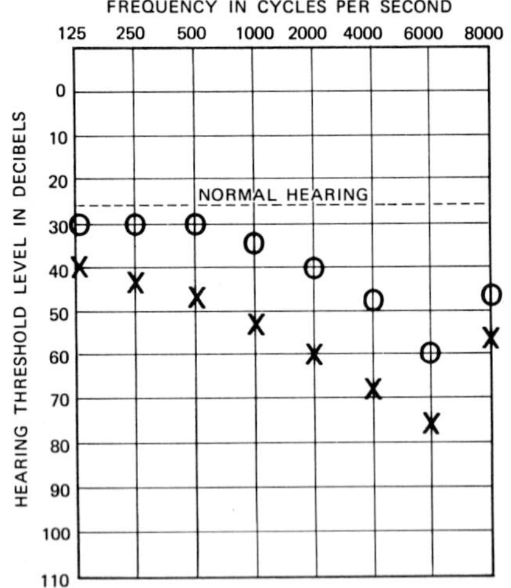

Figure 2.3. Typical audiogram of a patient with a sensorineural hearing loss. Diagnosis: noise-induced hearing loss. Compare with Figure 2.2. SRT = speech reception threshold; Discrim = word discrimination.

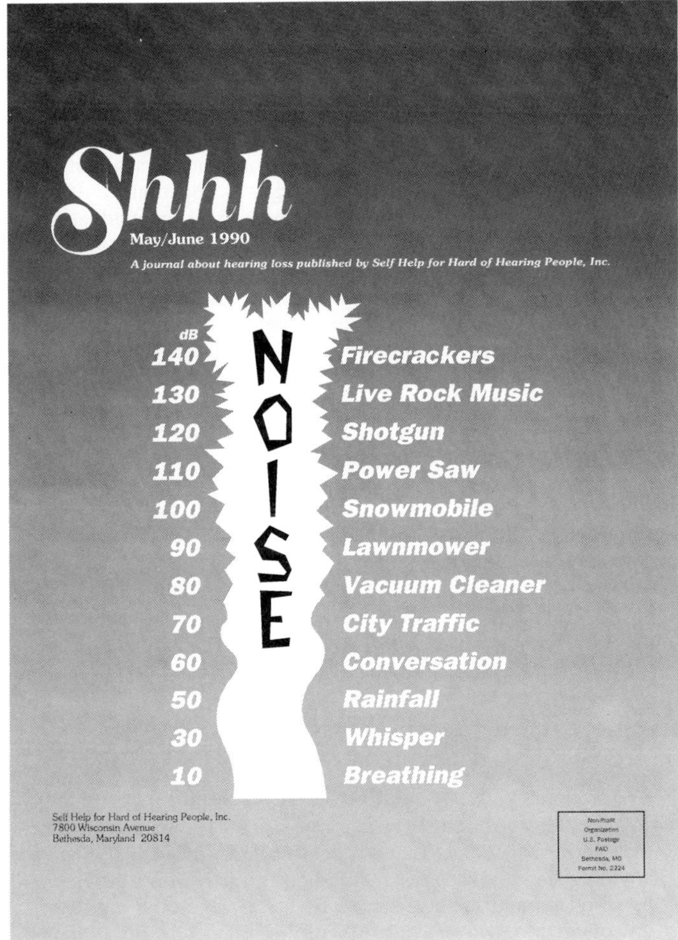

Figure 2.4. How loud is it. Noise intensities of everyday sounds expressed in decibels. Used with permission from SHHH—Self Help for Hard of Hearing People, Inc., 7800 Wisconsin Avenue, Bethesda, MD 20814.

is poor, and often recruitment can be demonstrated. The audiogram should differentiate presbycusis from noise-induced hearing loss. Historically, noise-induced hearing loss occurs in relatively young patients and is generally associated with significant noise exposure.

Life today is noisy. There is little question that prolonged unprotected exposure to loud noises (eg, aircraft engines) destroys cochlear hair cells and produces a sensorineural hearing impairment. But even the noises of everyday city living accumulate. Certainly some individuals are more sensitive, but everyone compromises their hearing acuity when they expose themselves to noise. Figure 2.4 shows the estimated noise exposures for several different common activities and provides a reference to noise intensities.

Any noise that hurts or leaves a ringing (tinnitus) or a temporary decrease in hearing is clearly damaging. The Occupational Safety and Health Administration has developed standards for the work environment, but they do not address the issues of lawn mowers, motorcycles, and loud music—the noises all are exposed to daily.

Patients only mildly affected should be encouraged to adapt to their disability and should be discouraged from purchasing hearing aids. Hearing aids are expensive (approximately $500 to $1000 at the time of this writing) and many are used for a limited time, then consigned to a bureau drawer. All hearing aids cause some distortion and they are only appreciated if they fit properly and the patient takes the time and energy to use them correctly. If the hearing loss worsens, a hearing aid evaluation by a qualified audiologist should be scheduled. The audiologist may recommend use of an aid, and if so, the patient should wear one on a trial basis. For patients who really need hearing aids, they restore the functionally deaf back to reasonable hearing. Sound is an extremely important part of human sensory input. Its loss causes a severe disability, and its restoration provides a tremendous improvement in the quality of life.

Case Studies: Presbycusis

A middle-aged couple visited my office. The woman stated that her husband was losing his hearing and was unable to hear anything she said. The patient did not feel there was a problem; he noted some difficulty hearing his wife, which did not seem to bother him. He had no difficulty talking with his golfing buddies. Physical examination was normal. The audiogram (see Fig. 2.2) showed a mild sensorineural hearing loss with good discrimination. Typically, the hearing loss is worse at high frequencies, so that female voices are more difficult to understand which may have somewhat explained any difficulty in hearing his wife. When the possibility of a hearing aid was discussed privately with the patient, he flatly refused to consider one. He stated that when he wanted to listen he had no difficulty. The patient was advised to return if his hearing worsened to a degree that he believed was causing a problem.

Another woman complained about her husband's hearing loss. Physical examination was normal, but the audiogram for this patient was different (see Fig. 2.3). The hearing worsened at each higher frequency and then became better at 8000 cps. The audiogram looked like a reverse check mark. This pattern is typical of a noise-induced hearing loss. Further history revealed this man was an avid duck hunter and trap shooter. He never wore protective ear covers and had always had quite a bit of high-pitched ringing in his ears after shooting. He was advised of the cause of his hearing loss and encouraged to wear both earplugs and earmuffs while shooting. He was also advised to return yearly for audiograms to determine if any progression in his hearing loss had occurred. He also declined to consider a hearing aid.

ACOUSTIC NEUROMA

Acoustic neuromas are benign tumors growing from the eighth cranial nerve, either in the internal auditory canal or at the cerebellar–pontine angle. Although they may be present in as many as 10% of the population at autopsy, they are detectable clinically in only 1 in 1000 patients. The tumors tend to occur in the fourth decade of life and later. Diverse presenting symptoms include hearing loss, vertigo, and occasionally facial paralysis. All patients with unexplained unilateral hearing loss, vertigo, or facial paralysis must be evaluated for an acoustic neuroma. With large tumors, other cranial nerves, especially the corneal branch of the fifth cranial nerve, may be involved. Audiograms usually show a sensorineural hearing loss with particularly poor discrimination or they may be near normal. A BERA reveals loss of waveform morphology and prolonged latencies of responses in the involved ear. Electronstagmography often shows a vestibular weakness of the involved ear. If acoustic neuroma is strongly suspected, a magnetic resonance imaging (MRI) scan with gadolinium should be performed to establish or rule out the diagnosis. Surgical excision is performed in all but elderly patients. This is often accomplished as a combined effort of head and neck surgeons and neurosurgeons.

A 19-year-old woman, status postresection of a left acoustic neuroma, returned for evaluation of a right acoustic neuroma. Her initial presentation was with a progressive sensorineural hearing loss, the left being worse than the right. In addition, over the preceding months she had developed a gait abnormality. She noted slurred speech and complained of headaches.

The initial left-side tumor resection left her with no auditory function and a facial paresis. Although the facial weakness was recovering, left promontory stimulation of the left ear revealed no cochlear nerve function. Her gait disturbance had been improving over time. Some sensorineural hearing remained intact on the right side. Figure 2.5 shows the MRI, revealing a large acoustic neuroma. The right-side acoustic neuroma was smaller than the tumor previously resected on the left side.

The patient underwent a suboccipital craniotomy as a combined neurosurgical/otologic procedure. The acoustic neuroma was resected. The cochlear and facial nerves were left intact and functioning.

Modern technology has introduced new treatments of complete deafness. Although there is no cure for complete or profound sensorineural hearing loss, there is a new rehabilitation option, cochlear implantation, available to those who no longer benefit from hearing aids. It is currently approved only for patients with bilateral profound deafness. An electrical device is implanted into the cochlea that allows direct stimulation of the neurons in the spiral ganglion. This stimulation signal is provided by an external device worn much like a Walkman® cassette player. Sound information is received and processed by the device and then transmitted to the implanted portion. The cochlear neurons are then stimulated electrically, causing the perception of sound. Although it does not restore normal hearing, patients relearn what the sounds signify, resulting in improved verbal communication.

For those with less severe hearing loss, significant advances have been made, and are yet to come, in modern hearing aids; better sound quality, smaller size, and, in some, remote controls to change loudness. A head and neck surgeon or qualified audiologist is best suited to advise patients regarding hearing rehabilitation options.

Ear disorders may lead to deafness, a devastating loss of a primary sense. Those deaf at birth or in infancy cannot hear anything so, it is difficult to learn the spoken language. Deaf individuals learn by sight; thus, spoken language is learned as a second language. Lip reading is difficult, even for those who become deaf as adults and it is extremely difficult for most prelingual deaf. Hence, signing is the primary communication form. The deaf community is effectively isolated. When they communicate to the rest of the world, it is through writing or an interpreter.

Deafness involves a sensory loss. The affected are those who are prevocationally deaf. In the United States there are 350,000 deaf persons, or 0.3% of the population.

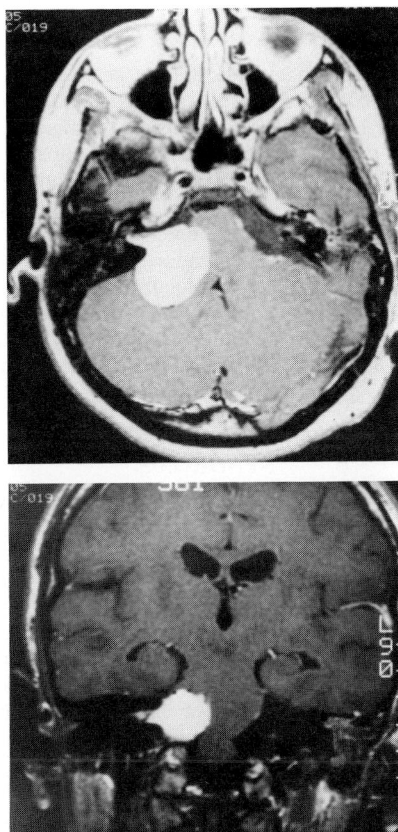

Figure 2.5. MRI scan with gadolinium. (A) T_1 axial view: right acoustic neuroma (3.0 × 3.5 cm) extending from internal auditory canal into cerebellar–pontine angle (note: brain stem compression). (B) T_1 coronal view. Again, note sizable right acoustic neuroma compressing brain stem and extending into the internal auditory canal.

In addition, many adults develop hearing impairments, some from infection, trauma, or tumors, but most from aging. Those who have severe-to-profound hearing loss are effectively deaf, and this has a large impact on their lives, including career changes and vocational training.

The deaf miss the pleasures of music, entertainment, and loved ones. Warning sounds used to protect and inform others, such as telephone rings and police sirens are not heard by deaf people. We normally live in a world of noise, a setting to which we are addicted. Absolute silence is hollow, lonely, distant, and isolated.

There are services available for the hearing impaired. Society provides courses in sign language. It provides interpreters to help communicate and take notes in school. There are also vocational rehabilitation programs. Flashing telephone and doorbell signalers are available to help the hearing impaired. Nonetheless, communication is an enormous problem, and physicians need to help the deaf individual when called on to do so. More can be learned about the deaf community, by visiting a school for the deaf or by contacting a social service agency that provides services to the deaf community.

TEMPOROMANDIBULAR JOINT SYNDROME

The temporomandibular joint (TMJ) syndrome is discussed in this section because patients with this condition frequently complain of ear pain. The TMJ, a sliding synovial joint, lies immediately in front of the bony external ear canal. Pain in this region is interpreted by patients as ear pain. The joint is affected, as are other synovial joints, by systemic arthritic conditions, including gout. Dental malocclusion, ill-fitting dentures, and psychologic stress are the most common causes of pain. Malocclusion causes stress on the joint with each mandibular excursion. Stress or tension often manifests as teeth clenching, excessive gum chewing, or bruxism (grinding the teeth, most commonly while asleep). The pain in the TMJ causes muscle spasm of the temporalis, masseter, pterygoid, digastric, tensor tympani, and at times the sternocleidomastoid muscles. In turn, this spasm causes more TMJ pain, and a cycle is established. The pain may be located primarily in front of the ear or it can be localized over the involved muscles. Spasm and pain in the temporalis muscle are often misdiagnosed as headache, especially migraine headache. Digastric and sternocleidomastoid muscle pain and spasm present in the neck and, frequently, these are not recognized as TMJ pain. Hearing loss, tinnitus, a feeling of fullness in the ear, and vertigo can also be symptoms of TMJ dysfunction. Temporomandibular joint pain may be the most commonly missed diagnosis in the head and neck region. Practitioners should become familiar with this disease; too many physicians repeatedly diagnose this as another problem, such as otitis externa or otitis media. Ear drops or antibiotics will not cure personal stress or dental malocclusion. The diagnosis of TMJ syndrome should be suspected in any patient who has complaints involving this region. Patients with this syndrome will indicate that the ear pain is anterior to the ear canal; no other pain presents here. Palpation over the TMJ

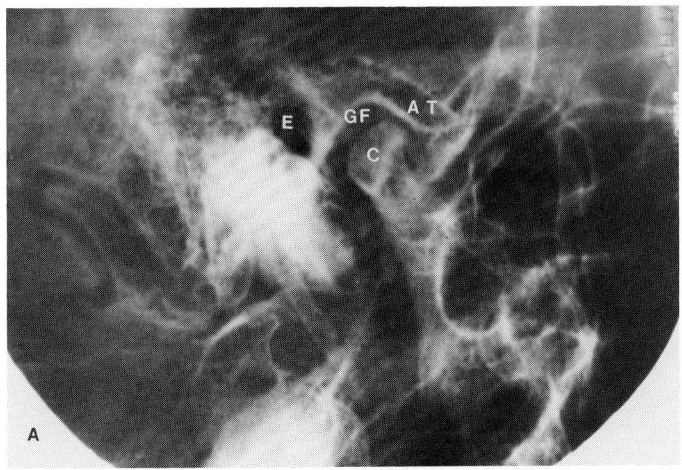

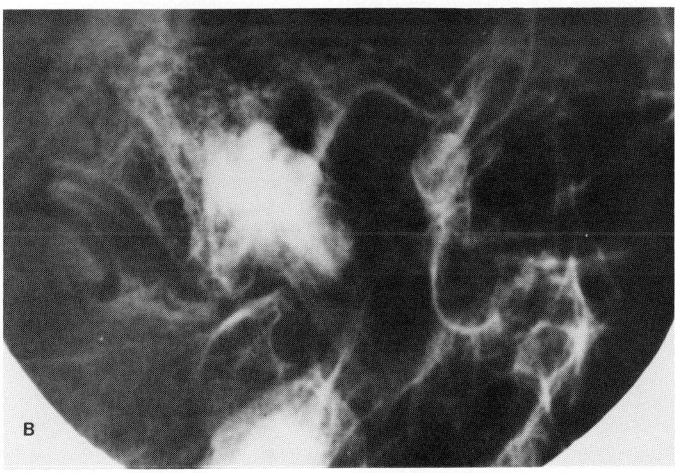

Figure 2.6. X rays from a patient with TMJ dysfunction. (A) Mouth closed and teeth in occlusion. (B) Mouth open. These X rays were read by the radiologist as normal. However, in the mouth-closed position, the condylar head appears pulled forward in the glenoid fossa. This is a common X ray finding in TMJ dysfunction. E = ear canal, GF = glenoid fossa, AT = articular tubercle, C = condyle.

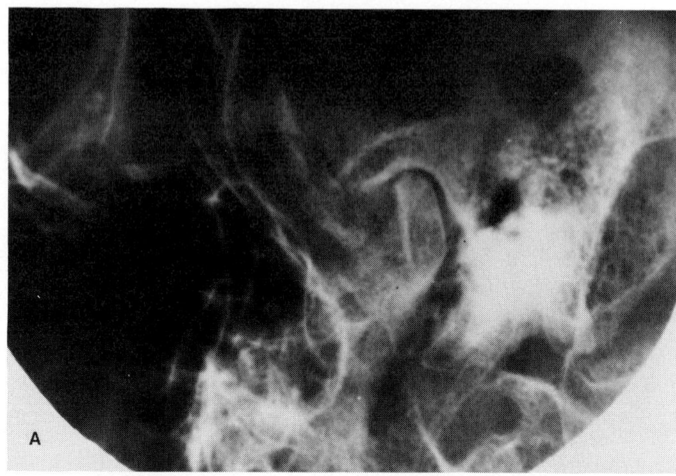

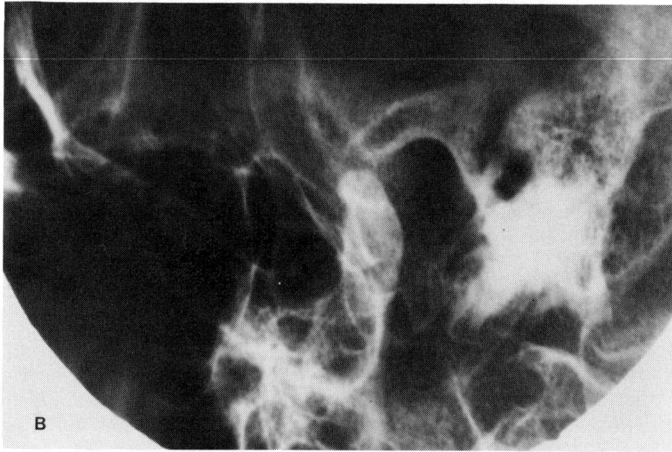

Figure 2.7. X rays from a patient with temporomandibular joint (TMJ) dysfunction. (A) Mouth closed. (B) Mouth open. In the mouth-open view, the condyle has slid anteriorly. This is not subluxation, but is commonly found in X rays of patients with and without TMJ dysfunction.

will elicit the pain, especially when the mouth is being opened and closed. Often the mandibular excursion is crooked and there is rather obvious malocclusion. The patient may have an anxious, distressed, or depressed expression, which is readily recognized by the sensitive physician. Often the patient can be shown the correlation between the TMJ pain and his or her tensions.

When evaluating TMJ dysfunction, X rays are useful to exclude destructive joint diseases. Oblique lateral views are taken so that the TMJs are not superimposed on one another. Two views are taken; one with the mouth closed and the teeth in normal occlusion and the second with the mouth widely open. Some physicians prefer TMJ tomograms and some prefer MRI scans, but plain films contain almost as much information, require less radiation exposure, and are cheaper. X rays are important to rule out arthritic bony changes. They will often show displacement of the condyle in the glenoid fossa caused by muscle spasm. Figures 2.6 and 2.7 show a right and left plain film TMJ series from two different patients with TMJ dysfunction. Neither shows arthritic changes, but both show subtle changes of TMJ muscle spasm. The MRI, although expensive, is the only study that will image the articular cartilage. It is certainly a superior study.

Malocclusive diseases are best treated by a dentist, orthodontist, or oral surgeon. Not all dentists are skilled with TMJ problems, and only those who are knowledgeable and interested will be helpful. Psychosomatic causes are best treated by the primary care physician, but if psychologic stresses are severe, the patient can be referred for psychotherapy.

The symptoms are best treated with analgesics (aspirin, NSAIDs, or acetaminophen) and muscle relaxants, such as diazepam. There are TMJ clinics in most major cities, and patients whose conditions are difficult to diagnose or treat can obtain more complete evaluation or treatment from such clinics.

Temporomandibular joint arthroscopy and arthroscopic surgery are sometimes recommended. Except in severe cases, they are not indicated because they may cause further damage and, in any case, are a needless expense. The legal profession has recognized this as a fruitful plaintiff's complaint. Lawyers may now refer postaccident "whiplash" patients to chiropractors and oral surgeons who seem to find TMJ problems where patient complaints did not previously exist. Once noted and treated the symptoms exacerbate, at least until a settlement is made, after which no one knows what happens to these individuals.

Case Study: Temporomandibular Joint Dysfunction

I received the following letter in response to a nationally distributed article and present it here (exactly as written) as an example of the complexity of TMJ dysfunction.

Dear Dr. Davidson:

I hope you won't mind my writing you directly. I saw an article on Tinnitus in the Health Fact News for April, that mentioned your name.

I am having such a time with noise in my right ear and its getting worse. I'm getting so nervous from it and its hard to concentrate at work. I live in fear this will start in the other ear and I don't know how I could stand it.

I first noticed the sound last December 19th when I was retiring for the night and the house was quiet. I thought I'd left the bathroom fluorescent light on as it was a hum or drone just as my ear now has. (I don't know if this could be a clue or not, but I had a gold crown put on a lower right tooth on December 18th.)

At first, I only heard the sound at night, but by late February it had worsened and I saw my doctor about it. He asked me to describe the noise and when I said it was like the sound of a fluorescent light "hum or sing" or like the dial tone on a telephone, he said "that's 60 cycles—you have fluid in your Eustachian tube." He began treatment with an injection of Decadon or (Decadron) and a prescription for Historodrix. [I do not know what Historodrix is. Au.] I have reactions to so many drugs and after four days became ill so he gave me Rondec tablets. I had the same reaction to that after a couple days and then along with the original noise my ear started to ring also. It is now two different sounds in that ear.

I asked my Dr. if he would send me to an ear specialist. The closest is Duluth, Mn. at the Duluth Clinic. I saw this Dr. on March 25. He looked in my ear just as my M.D. had and said there was no fluid in the Eustachian tube. (?) I had an Audio, AC only and Speech Audiometry Dis. The Dr. said my hearing was excellent, even exceptional! He had no idea what the problem could be. He pressed on my jaw joints and could cause tinnitus, but wasn't sure that was my problem. He suggested watching to see if I grit my teeth, etc. During the audio test the lady who gave the test could match up the ringing noise with her equipment, but not the droning buzz I hear.

I mentioned the gold crown to this Dr. and said it was high at first but had it corrected in January. Since then an upper right tooth had broken off and the Otolaryngologist said to see my dentist next. I only saw this Dr. about 10 minutes. He prescribed a mild dosage of Valium as muscle relaxant in case I was clenching my jaws. My M.D. won't even write a prescription for Valium. He is really against it.

After my dentist returned from his vacation I was able to see him April 16th. The cracked tooth (also on the right side) turned out to be abscessed and dead. He extracted the tooth and said the abscess looked almost like a cyst. We were both sure now that the ear noise would stop, but as of this writing it's even louder.

My life is turning into a nightmare. I was sure the Ear Specialist would have done more diagnostic tests, but maybe there are no others? He suggested sleeping with an F-M radio dial set between two stations, but I'm leaving that as a last resort. He said there are devices similar to hearing-aids to put in the ear to try to counteract the noise, but because my hearing is so good he didn't want to do that.

I wake up some mornings with a vague ache in that ear and in the bone behind the ear. It always feels heavy now and a sort of tightness or stiffness deep in there when I yawn. It just feels if I could "pop" it when I yawn it would be alright again.

We live up here in Minnesota in a small logging village (Pop. 500) and my M.D. is forty miles away.

Can you give me any suggestion? I would deeply appreciate any advice you might have.

I hope you don't mind my writing to you personally, but I am getting desperate with this problem. It seems there must be an answer somewhere! I have even wondered if a person could be surgically deafened to stop the noise?

Thank you for anything you may have to suggest!

Sincerely,
Mrs. E.L.D.

P.S. I am 51 years old. Almost thru Menopause and no problems there. My last blood pressure check in February was 110/82. I don't smoke, drink or use aspirin. I use CoTylenol occasionally if I have a cold. I drink approx. two cups of decaffeinated coffee per day. I do have a lot of sinus postnasal drip, have had for years, but no pain. Just have to blow my nose a lot each day.

I keep wondering if that gold crown could in any way be picking up an electric signal or something? It sounds odd, but at this point you want to check anything that might bring relief.

Used with the written permission of the patient.

In view of the normal audiogram this patient's problem is most likely due to TMJ dysfunction. I advised her of this and referred her to a physician in her area who was knowledgeable about TMJ disease.

OTALGIA

Otalgia (ear pain) is a common complaint, and although the cause is sometimes obvious, it can just as often be obscure. There are a multitude of causes of ear pain, and unless a systematic approach is followed, important diagnoses may be missed. Table 2.2 describes the differential diagnosis for ear pain. These areas noted in Table 2.2

Table 2.2 Differential Diagnosis for Ear Pain

A. External auditory canal
   1. Auricular hemotoma
   2. Foreign body in the ear canal
   3. Obstructive cerumen
   4. Otitis externa
   5. Malignant otitis externa
   6. External auditory canal tumor
B. Middle ear
   1. Acute otitis media
   2. Bullous myringitis or a mycoplasmal infection of the tympanic membrane
   3. Chronic otitis media
   4. Middle ear tumor
C. Temporomandibular joint (TMJ) dysfunction
D. Referred pain from an inflammatory or neoplastic lesion
   1. Nasopharynx
   2. Tonsil
   3. Base of tongue
   4. Larynx
   5. Pharynx and hypopharynx

are evaluated by direct examination, palpation, mirror examination, endoscopy, cultures, and biopsies.

HEARING LOSS AND TINNITUS

Hearing loss is a common complaint. Occasionally patients complain of a ringing or hissing noise (tinnitus). Tinnitus is normally high-pitched; a similar sound can be heard by holding a seashell or a cup over an ear. To some, the sound is a buzzing or hissing, but to others it is a more distinct ringing. It seems that when the ear loses its hearing sensitivity, the brain somehow substitutes its own noise. Not everyone with hearing loss complains of tinnitus, but for those who do, it has a direct relationship; that is, the greater the hearing loss, the greater the tinnitus. There are now ways of treating tinnitus, but first it should be recognized that it is usually a symptom of hearing loss. The hearing loss should be diagnosed and, if there is no direct treatment, the tinnitus treated. Occasionally, tinnitus has a low-pitched quality—even the physician can hear it with the stethoscope. This type is caused by vascular noise. It may be a bruit or murmur in the carotid artery or a chemodectoma, also called a glomus tumor, in the middle ear. These patients should be evaluated by a head and neck surgeon. The differential diagnosis for hearing loss is shown in Table 2.3.

Table 2.3 Differential Diagnosis for Hearing Loss

A. External auditory canal
    1. Cerumen (wax)
    2. Foreign body
    3. Otitis externa
    4. Exostosis
    5. Tumor
B. Middle ear
    1. Acute otitis media
    2. Chronic otitis media
    3. Serous otitis media
    4. Tympanic membrane perforation
    5. Otosclerosis
    6. Ossicular discontinuity or fixation
    7. Round window rupture (barotrauma)
    8. Tumor
C. Inner ear
    1. Presbycusis
    2. Noise-induced hearing loss
    3. Meniere's disease
    4. Otosclerosis
    5. Ototoxic drug-induced hearing loss
    6. Labyrinthitis
       a. Serous: following trauma, ear surgery, or infectious otitis media
       b. Viral, such as mumps, measles, and so forth
       c. Bacterial
       d. Toxic
    7. Congenital sensorineural hearing loss
    8. Trauma
    9. Neurosyphilis
   10. Vascular insufficiency
D. Central nervous system
    1. Cerebrovascular accident
    2. Acoustic neuroma
    3. Brain tumor
    4. Psychiatric disorder

Hearing Loss Evaluation

Any patient with hearing loss should have a history taken. Questions should address onset, duration, severity, associated symptoms (eg, tinnitus, vertigo, ear infections, surgery), unilateral or bilateral, noise exposure, ototoxic medication exposure, and other medial conditions. The information discovered during the questioning will serve to direct the physician in further examination and testing. Physical examination should include the auricle, external auditory canal, tympanic membrane, the Weber and the Rinne tuning fork tests, and facial nerve function. One should look for evidence of infection, cholesteatoma, perforation, scarring, cerumen impaction, or neoplasm. Once the physical examination has been completed, an audiogram should be performed using air conduction, bone conduction, and speech discrimination testing. Based on the findings of the audiogram, history, and examination, a diagnosis is usually established. However, further testing may occasionally be indicated to rule out retro cochlear or central dysfunction.

In patients with asymmetric symptoms of tinnitus, or sensorineural hearing loss, a BERA may be necessary to track the electric nerve signal produced from cochlear stimulation from the cochlea to the brain stem. A clicking sound is presented to the ear at an appropriate volume to generate a response. Then the EEG response is measured and averaged over approximately 1000 to 2000 clicks. Changes in wave form, pattern, and latency of recognized waves are evaluated to determine whether the deficit is peripheral or central in nature.

VERTIGO

Vertigo is a feeling that the world is spinning around. People with extreme vertigo feel nauseous, often vomit, and talk about lying down and holding onto the carpet to keep from falling off the earth. Many patients complain of dizziness rather than of a true whirling sensation. A whirling sensation is usually associated with some identifiable etiology. The patient who complains of being dizzy may have a clear-cut and identifiable significant disorder, but often the diagnosis may remain somewhat obscure. Dizziness takes a long time to evaluate, and may require a complete history and a physical and laboratory examination. Time spent on the history will help direct the physician in decisions regarding testing and treatment. Failure to be thorough will result in missed diagnoses. Physicians in different specialties have different experiences with vertigo. A triage officer at a Veterans Administration hospital, for example, may cite the leading causes of vertigo as cardiac arrhythmia and orthostatic hypotension. A neurologist might consider multiple sclerosis the most common cause, while a head and neck surgeon might believe that Meniere's disease or vestibular neuronitis is most common. To a general practitioner most causes are idiopathic or functional. Each of these physicians reflects the nature of his or her own practice.

Table 2.4 is an evaluation for each of my patients who complain of dizziness; it can be used as a guide for developing personal approaches. Figure 2.8 provides an algorithm for differential diagnosis.

Treatment
The treatment of vertigo often falls closer to the art than to the science of medicine. It sometimes seems that all of the physician's energy has been used in merely obtaining the history, conducting the labo-

Table 2.4 Work-Up for Vertigo History

A. *History*
 1. Vertigo (what does the patient mean by dizziness?)
    a. Onset
    b. Intensity
    c. Duration
    d. Association with nausea and vomiting
    e. Feeling of faintness or loss of consciousness
 2. Hearing loss
 3. Tinnitus
 4. Feeling of fullness in ear
 5. History of ear pain, infection, or surgery
 6. Recent illness
 7. Current medications
 8. Previous neurologic disorders (transient ischemic attack, stroke, multiple sclerosis, migraine headache)
B. *Examination*
 1. Hearing (tuning forks)
 2. Otoscopic
 3. Ophthalmic (to include extraocular movements, examination for nystagmus, and retinoscopy)
 4. Cranial nerves, with particular attention to nerves 3, 4, 5 (especially corneal branch), 6, 7, 9, and 10
 5. Neck examination (to recognize carotid artery disease) and range of motion
 6. Blood pressure (to consider hypertension and orthostatic changes
 7. Pulse (to diagnose arrhythmia)
 8. Neurologic (to exclude neurologic disease, especially multiple sclerosis and a cerebrovascular accident)
C. *Laboratory tests*
 1. Complete blood cell count (to rule out anemia)
 2. Electrolytes (to detect any imbalance)
 3. Calcium (to detect hypercalcemia)
 4. Tetraiodothyronine (to detect hypothyroidism)
 5. FTA-ABS, T4, and TSH (to rule out tertiary syphilis)
 6. Cholesterol and triglycerides (to detect hyperlipoproteinemia)
 7. Tests for diabetes and reactive hypoglycemia
 8. Electrocardiogram with rhythm strip (to diagnose any cardiac disease in elderly patients or with history suggestive of cardiac dysfunction)
 9. Audiogram and tympanogram (to evaluate hearing as well as evaluate type of loss) and BERA (to evaluate retrocochlear sensorineural hearing loss (see Fig. 1.9)
 10. Electronystagmogram (to evaluate labyrinthine function). This test measures gaze nystagmus, spontaneous nystagmus, positional nystagmus, and response to caloric irrigation. It is extremely useful to identify labyrinthine disease and also helps localize lesions in either the labyrinth, the acoustic nerve, or the central nervous system

(continued)

Table 2.4 Continued

11. MRI scan with gadolinium of internal auditory canal indicated when acoustic neuroma, cerebellar-pontine angle tumor, multiple sclerosis or other central problem suspected
12. X rays of the cervical spine. The cervical spine is closely connected to the labyrinth via a vestibulospinal reflex arc. Cervical spine disease can cause vertigo and hence this must be evaluated

D. *Differential diagnosis* (also see Figure 2.8)
This is not intended as an exhaustive differential plan, but rather to provide some insight into the different diseases that can cause vertigo. If the investigator is persistent a diagnosis can be made in over 90% of vertiginous patients.
  1. Ear
    a. Acute otitis media
    b. Serous otitis media
    c. Chronic otitis media
    d. Perilymph fistula
      i. Trauma
      ii. Poststapedectomy
      iii. Barotrauma (round window rupture)
    e. Labyrinthitis
      i. Serous
      ii. Bacterial
      iii. Viral
      iv. Toxic
    f. Meniere's disease
    g. Vestibular neuronitis
    h. Benign positional vertigo
    i. Acoustic neuroma or other cerebellar–pontine angle tumor
  2. Central nervous system
    a. Stroke (cerebrovascular accident)
    b. Transient ischemic attacks
    c. Multiple sclerosis
    d. Neurosyphilis
    e. Meningitis or encephalitis
    f. Migraine (posterior fossa)
  3. Neck
    a. Cervical arthritis
    b. Carotid artery stenosis
    c. Vertebral–basilar artery insufficiency
    d. Subclavian steal syndrome
    e. TMJ disease
  4. Metabolic disorders
    a. Hyper- or hypoglycemia
    b. Hyper- or hypothyroidism
    c. Electrolyte imbalance
    d. Hypercalcemia
    e. Anemia
    f. Polycythemia
    g. Leukemia
    h. Allergy

Table 2.4 Continued

5. Infections
    a. Influenza
    b. Herpes zoster
    c. Measles
    d. Mumps
    e. Other viral illnesses
6. Drugs
    a. Streptomycin
    b. Kanamycin
    c. Gentamicin
    d. Diazepam
    e. Sedatives
    f. Opiates
    g. Alcohol
    h. Neuroleptics
    i. Aspirin
    j. Nicotine
    k. Caffeine
7. Cardiac problems
    a. Arrhythmia
    b. Hypertension
    c. Hypotension
    d. Poor cardiac output

BERA = brain stem evoked response audiometry; FTA-ABS = fluorescent treponema antibody; T_4 = thyroxine; TSH = thyroid stimulating hormone.

ratory examination, and reaching a reasonable diagnosis, and there is none left for creative therapy.

Specific causes of vertigo are treated. Bacterial labyrinthitis is a severe disease and obviously must be treated with antibiotics, usually in the hospital. It is often considered a surgical emergency and cause for labyrinthectomy to prevent spread of infection to the central nervous system. Patients with vascular problems are referred to specialists in vascular diseases, and those with neurologic diseases to neurologists. Otologic diseases causing vertigo are appropriately the province of the head and neck surgeon. The remainder—and actual majority of cases—are treated by primary care physicians, emergency department physicians, and head and neck surgeons. Although some physicians have elaborate therapeutic regimens, a simple approach is equally effective: Phenothiazines are the mainstay of treatment, and promethazine hydrochloride is as effective as any. For mild cases, 25 mg promethazine can be taken orally every 6 hours. For some patients, diazepam is useful alone or in combination with promethazine. For moderately intense attacks, IV promethazine is indicated to stabilize the vertigo, after which oral or rectal suppositories can be used. Patients with severe cases are frequently dehydrated and need IV fluids. Promethazine is given IV, frequently with diazepam.

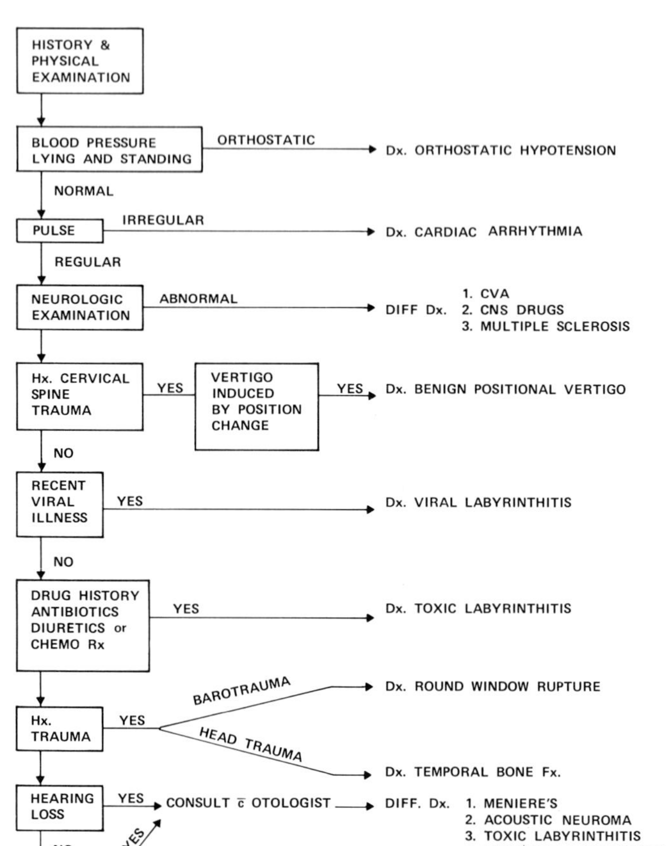

Figure 2.8.   Algorithm for the diagnosis of vertigo.

Alternatively, 0.5 mg to 1.5 mg IV droperidol is effective in those patients unresponsive to diazepam. Promethazine should not be given in conjunction with the droperidol therapy. Hospitalization is often necessary. Intractable labyrinthine vertigo can be treated surgically, with cure rates approaching 90% to 95%.

Many patients will request medication to combat motion sickness and a number of medications are useful. The first choice of drug for air sickness or seasickness is usually a nonprescription medicine such as Dramamine® or Meclizine. An effective prescription is Antivert. These are effective and, although they cause some sleepiness, tend to be mild. If the patient complains of motion sickness symptoms with very mild stimulation, such as flying in a modern jet or a long trip in a car, the reason may be psychologic. For these conditions, diazepam is effective, because it allays the patient's anxiety and it is also an effective vestibular sedative.

The most difficult cases are those people with sensitive vestibular systems who, nevertheless, occasionally wish to go boating in ocean waters where they are exposed to intense vestibular stimulation. Oral promethazine is extremely effective in these situations; 25 mg can be taken the evening before boating, and should be repeated approximately 1 to 1.5 hours before embarking. All of the phenothiazines have a long onset time; that is, they are not effective for at least 1 to 1.5 hours, and they also have a long half-life. Therefore, the promethazine taken 12 hours earlier will still have some vestibular sedating effect when the patient embarks. Many patients do not like to take the evening dose of promethazine and simply begin with the first dose 1.5 hours before going aboard. Unfortunately, such a dose will put most people to sleep. If it is possible to board the boat and sleep for the first several hours and allow their vestibular systems to adjust to the rocking of the boat while they are asleep, many patients will require little or no additional medicine. If any is needed, the original dose can be repeated every 6 hours. If it is important that the person be alert and functional at the beginning of the trip, it will be necessary to give some stimulant to counteract the sedative effects of the promethazine, such as 25 mg promethazine with 25 mg ephedrine, both to be taken orally at least 1.5 hours before boarding and not to be repeated more than once every 6 hours.

Another drug combination that has been popular with many sailors is 0.5 mg scopolamine with 2.5 to 10 mg dextroamphetamine. This combination tends to be less sedating than promethazine and ephedrine. Another popular medication with many sailors is scopolamine supplied as a sticky patch to be placed on the skin behind the ear (Transderm-Scōp). The scopalamine is absorbed slowly and is reputed to be effective for periods of 2 to 3 days. Its side effects—which some find irritating—include a dry mouth and pupillary dilatation. For some, the side effects are intolerable. It is, at the time of this writing, the most popular prescription treatment for motion sickness. It is contraindicated in the geriatric population.

Many times "on-board physicians" are asked to treat motion sickness once it has occurred. In such circumstances, the previous recommendations are usually not effective. Promethazine given intramuscularly or as a rectal suppository is effective. If this fails, IV fluids combined with promethazine or droperidol can be required.

Individual head and neck surgeons organize their thoughts and their therapies regarding vertigo differently. Table 2.5 outlines an alternative differential diagnosis, evaluation, and treatment of vertigo.

Table 2.5 Differential Diagnosis, Evaluation, and Treatment of Vertigo

---

I. *Vestibular Neuronitis*
   A. Presenting signs and symptoms: acute onset of severe vertigo may be episodic and may be associated with preexistent upper respiratory infection, spontaneous nystagmus, and normal hearing
   B. Etiology: probably viral neuronitis, with degeneration of Scarpa's ganglion and peripheral neurons
   C. Laboratory tests: reduced vestibular response (RVR) in affected ear found on caloric testing; normal CNS examination
   D. Treatment:
       1. Symptomatic: rehydration
       2. Drugs:
           a. Meclizine, 12.5–25 mg/d po, divided into equal doses given q4h
           b. Dimenhydrinate, 25–50 mg pp or IM q4–6h
           c. Diazepam, 5–10 mg IM or IV q4–6h
           d. Promethazine, 25–50 mg IM or po q6–8h
   E. Prognosis: patient usually improves over a 1-month period; however, there may be exacerbations for as long as 1 year. Canal paresis persists
II. *Acute labyrinthitis (sudden hearing loss)*
   A. Presenting signs and symptoms: acute onset of severe vertigo associated with hearing loss (mild to profound) and spontaneous nystagmus
   B. Etiology: probably virally induced cochleolabyrinthitis (widespread, with damage to inner ear structures)
   C. Laboratory tests:
       1. Audiogram: sensorineural hearing loss
       2. Electronystagmography: reduced vestibular response must be evaluated for CNS disease
       3. Other tests:
           a. Mastoid tomograms
           b. VDRL, FTA-ABS
           c. T_3 (triiodothyronine), T_4 (thyroxine)
           d. Complete blood count, glucose tolerance test
           e. Sedimentation rate, cholesterol, triglycerides, ANA (antinuclear antibody), and RF (rheumatoid factor)
   D. Treatment:
       1. Symptomatic: rehydration
       2. Drugs: prednisone, 60–80 mg/d, tapering dose over 3 weeks (if not contraindicated)
   E. Prognosis: usually dizziness subsides with time. If patient has U-shaped or upward-sloping audiogram, there is a good chance for recovery
III. *Meniere's Disease*
   A. Presenting signs and symptoms:
       1. Attacks of episodic vertigo, pressure in ear, hearing fluctuation, roaring tinnitus
       2. Nystagmus (only during acute attack)

Table 2.5 Continued

---

      3. Low-frequency sensorineural hearing loss
      4. Normal findings between episodes (early in the disease)
  B. Etiology: secondary to endolymphatic hydrops
      1. Idiopathic
      2. Following temporal bone fracture
      3. Following meningitis
      4. Following sudden hearing loss (from mumps, etc.)
  C. Laboratory tests: document low-frequency hearing loss by audiometry. Same evaluation as for acute labyrinthitis (II-C)
  D. Treatment: same as for vestibular neuronitis (I-D). Reduce salt to 1500 mg/d and caffeine intake, food additives. Give diuretics if symptoms do not respond to dietary changes alone. Surgery may be indicated if vertigo becomes incapacitating
  E. Prognosis: Variable. Symptoms may stop altogether or be episodic and eventually cause total sensorineural hearing loss with severe disabling vertigo. Disease is bilateral in 20%–40%

IV. *Benign positional vertigo (BPV), cupulolithiasis*
  A. Presenting signs and symptoms:
      1. Attacks of true vertigo occurring with the patient in supine position and typically with involved ear down
      2. Latency of 5–6 seconds before vertigo begins
      3. Nystagmus is generally rotatory toward the down ear
      4. Fatigues with repeated testing
      5. Normal hearing; may be without trauma
      6. Attacks last seconds to minutes
  B. Etiology: degenerative otoliths from utricular macula drift by gravity and become embedded in cupula of posterior canal crista
  C. Laboratory tests: Positional testing in office. Electronystagmography demonstrates positional rotatory nystagmus, delay in onset, fatiguing, fixation, or suppression. No CNS signs are present
  D. Treatment:
      1. Advise patient to repeatedly assume the positions causing vertigo; provide information and reassurance. Vestibular conditioning exercises will speed recovery in most patients
      2. Cawthorne exercises (vestibular conditioning exercises)
      3. Surgery: singular nerve section, or vestibular nerve section
  E. Prognosis: usually subsides with time, especially in young patients. If present longer than 6 months, consider surgery

V. *Acoustic neurinoma (Schwannoma)*
  A. Presenting signs and symptoms:
      1. Unilateral, progressive, sensorineural hearing loss (typically high frequency)
      2. Tinnitus in affected ear

(continued)

Table 2.5 Continued

---

      3. Mild disequilibrium, which may mimic Meniere's disease
      4. Occasional pain or pressure in affected ear (not always present)
  B. Etiology: Schwann cell or eighth nerve tumor (superior vestibular nerve most common origin); may be intracanalicular or extend into the cerebellar–pontine angle and compress the brain stem
  C. Laboratory tests:
      1. Brain stem-evoked-response audiometry (BERA) (see Figure 1.9): delay in wave V must be compared with other ear; latency wave V greater than 0.02 ms is significant
      2. Electronystagmography: reduced vestibular response
      3. Audiometry: poor speech discrimination in 50%–60%, tone decay, high-frequency sensorineural hearing loss, reflex decay
      4. MRI scan with gadolinium of internal auditory canals and cerebellar–pontine angles is study of choice
      5. If MRI unavailable then high resolution CT scan with contrast
  D. Treatment
      1. Surgical removal
      2. If patient is older than 70 years, some consideration should be given to observing the patient and not operating unless symptoms necessitate surgical decompression
  E. Prognosis: excellent if operated on early. However, there is a good chance of dead ear resulting from removal of tumor. Facial nerve paralysis may occur from removal of larger tumors. Untreated, they cause death by brain-stem compression
VI. *Neuro-otosyphilis (congenital or late)*
  A. Presenting signs and symptoms: fluctuating sensorineural hearing loss, episodic vertigo, tinnitus; may be bilateral. Other stigmata of syphilis may be present. Positive Hennebert's sign (pressure in the ear canal causes nystagmus)
  B. Etiology: endolymphatic hydrops, periostitis, obliterative endarteritis
  C. Laboratory tests:
      1. VDRL is negative in 70% of patients
      2. FTA-ABS: false-positive in 6%, false-negative in 5%. May be positive in collagen-vascular disorders, autoimmune hemolytic anemias, cirrhosis, and occasionally pregnancy. Test must be repeated if + 1
  D. Treatment
      1. Penicillin G (crystalline), 2–4 million U IV q4h for 10 days

or

      2. Penicillin G (procaine), 60,000 U/d IM for 25 days

or

      3. Penicillin G (benzathine), 2.4 million U/wk IM for 3 weeks

Table 2.5 Continued

---

or
    4. Tetracycline hydrochloride, 500 mg po q6h for 30 days
or
    5. Erythromycin, 500 mg po q6h, with probenecid, 0.5 g q6 for 30 days, and prednisone, 40–60 mg/d po for 3 weeks and ten 5–10 mg/d for maintenance
  E. Prognosis: often exacerbates, requiring boost in steroid therapy or retreatment

VII. *Inner ear fistula (round window or oval window)*
  A. Presenting signs and symptoms:
    1. Sudden onset of mild, moderate, or severe hearing loss (may fluctuate) associated with vertigo or ataxia
    2. Most often related to barotrauma, exertion, trauma, or surgery
    3. Spontaneous nystagmus
    4. Positional vertigo
  B. Etiology: small leakage of perilymph out of inner ear via round window membrane or oval window
  C. Laboratory tests:
    1. Fistula test positive
    2. Electronystagmography: may be reduced vestibular response, positional nystagmus, positive fistual test
    3. Audiometry: sensorineural hearing loss
  D. Treatment: strict bed rest for 5 days. Surgical exploration and repair of fistula
  E. Prognosis: good for recovery from vertigo, poor for hearing improvement

VIII. *Suppurative labyrinthitis*
  A. Presenting signs and symptoms:
    1. Foul-smelling otorrhea
    2. History of chronic otitis media or cholesteatoma
    3. Severe vertigo or dizziness
    4. Fever
  B. Etiology: bacterial invasion of inner ear (commonly *Pseudomonas*)
  C. Laboratory tests:
    1. Gram stain
    2. Culture and sensitivity tests
    3. CT scan of temporal bones
    4. Lumbar puncture
    5. Audiometry
  D. Treatment
    1. Hospitalization
    2. IV antibiotics
    3. Mastoidectomy and possible labyrinthectomy
  E. Prognosis: if diagnosed early enough, the condition may be cured with medical or surgical therapy. Otherwise can lead to dead ear, meningitis, or brain abscess

---

Table courtesy of Jeffrey Harris, M.D.

FACIAL PARALYSIS

Facial paralysis is a relatively common problem. If permanent, it is tremendously incapacitating. The human face is an animated structure, and when it becomes paralyzed, the animation is lost. The face droops and appears grotesque. The eye can no longer close and may dry out. The resultant corneal ulcerations cause blindness. Saliva drools from the corner of the sagging mouth. Many aspects of an individual's social life are seriously compromised. In children, facial paralysis may be congenital, traumatic, occasionally neoplastic, or, rarely, caused by ear infection. Paralysis in young adults is often idiopathic. Other causes, such as brain tumor, otologic disease, and parotid neoplasms, must be excluded. Temporal bone fractures can cause facial paralysis, but the most common causes remain idiopathic. Idiopathic facial paralysis is called Bell's palsy, but facial paralysis should not be presumed idiopathic and should not be called Bell's palsy until a complete work-up has been conducted, including a complete history, and a physical examination that encompasses an otoscopic examination, palpation of the parotid gland, and a full cranial nerve examination. Each of the branches of the facial nerve must be tested. The greater superficial petrosal nerve leaves the facial nerve intracranially at the geniculate ganglion. It innervates the lacrimal gland, and its function is measured by the Schirmer test. The facial nerve supplies sensation to the posterior external auditory canal wall, which is easily tested. The stapedial reflex is measured by tympanometry. The chorda tympani innervates the taste buds on the anterior two thirds of the tongue and stimulates salivary flow from the submandibular gland. Both can be tested. The peripheral branches of the facial nerve exit at the stylomastoid foramen, course through the parotid gland, and innervate the facial musculature. As they function they can be observed and compared with the function on the contralateral side of the face. If the face is paralyzed, electric nerve-conduction studies are necessary to document facial nerve conduction, degeneration, regeneration, and function. Although CT is the examination of choice for many temporal bone inflammatory illnesses such as chronic otitis media, the facial nerve is best seen with MRI and gadolinium enhancement. Figure 2.9 summarizes these tests.

With facial nerve paralysis, the eye may close poorly and the lacrimal secretion may be reduced. Because of the decreased lacrimal secretion, the cornea can dry and ulcerate in 12 to 24 hours. Prophylaxis should be started immediately by supplying the patient with artificial tears to be used every hour and as needed for burning or drying. This applies to waking hours; at night, patients need a moisture chamber made with a properly shaped piece of plastic wrap that can be taped (with nonallergenic paper tape) to the eyebrow, nose, lower eyelid, and cheekbone. This mask will enclose and protect the eye at night, and for some patients, it is also necessary during the day. LacriLube® (Allergan) or a similar nonantibiotic, nonsteroidal oint-

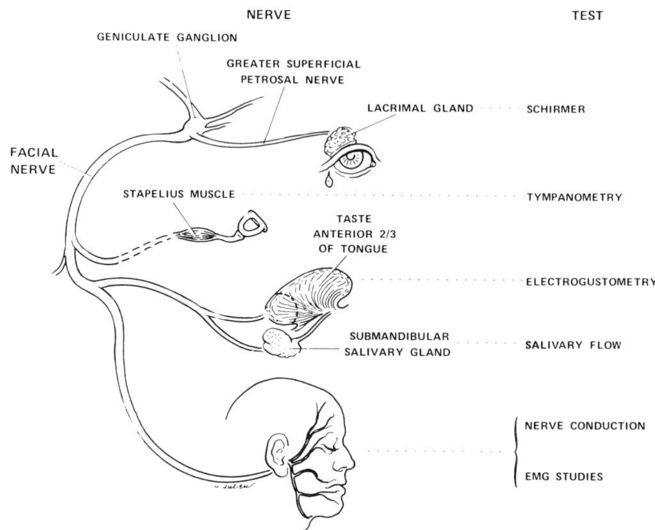

Figure 2.9. Facial nerve function. Drawing summarizing facial nerve function and tests currently available to assess each function. This type of testing helps confirm specific diagnoses and also helps localize the site of a lesion.

ment should be placed in the eye at night before applying the moisture chamber.

If a complete work-up fails to elucidate a specific etiology for the paralysis, a diagnosis of idiopathic facial paralysis (Bell's palsy) can be made. This paralysis can affect any age group. It is more common in pregnant women. Sometimes, it is related to a viral upper RTI infection. Usually, it has a sudden onset without other major symptoms. Treatment is controversial. Many physicians in the United States treat the condition with steroid therapy for 1 or 2 weeks; however, evidence is lacking to support this therapy. Roughly 85% of patients recover their facial function fully, although a small number develop a permanent total paralysis. All patients with a total paralysis must be studied with nerve conduction testing. If the nerve is electrically nonconductive, that patient's prognosis is poor and surgical decompression of the facial nerve in the temporal bone will improve the outcome. Surgery is indicated for fewer than 5% of patients with facial paralysis. Traumatic facial paralysis must be evaluated carefully. In many cases, surgery is necessary to repair or decompress the nerve in the temporal bone.

The social and the physiologic handicap of complete facial paralysis is immense. These patients are at constant risk that the eye will dry, and they drool constantly. A paralyzed face may seem grotesque to others, and people so affected often become social recluses. Techniques are available for facial rehabilitation. A nerve graft is used if a segment of the facial nerve is destroyed. If the proximal nerve is destroyed but the peripheral neuromuscular system is intact, the hypoglossal nerve can be anastomosed to the facial nerve. This provides tone and, with biofeedback training, volitional movement to the face. When the distal nerve or neuromuscular system, or both, are sacrificed, as in radical parotid gland neoplasm resections, a whole new nerve and muscle system must be provided. An operation called a temporalis muscle sling does this by freeing the temporalis muscle from the zygoma to the midline of the scalp. The muscle is divided into long, thin strips, which are threaded about the eyes, mouth, and face. These produce a dynamic sling that, although not perfect, is a tremendous improvement over a totally paralyzed face. All the procedures mentioned are performed by head and neck surgeons.

CHAPTER 3

The Nose

The nose and paranasal sinuses are the causes of many major and minor ailments. Their anatomy and function are poorly understood by most. The nose and sinuses can be involved in congenital abnormalities, tumors, infections, trauma, and metabolic disease.

EPISTAXIS

The bloody nose is a common emergency problem. The majority are spontaneous, with no identifiable cause, although many are traumatic. Nonobvious causes cannot be overlooked, such as hemophilia, other coagulopathies, leukemia, or intranasal neoplasms. As usual, a complete history is taken. Use of aspirin, NSAIDs, or sodium warfarin ingestion should be ascertained. Children and many adults often cause bleeding by nose picking. A pubertal male may have an angiofibroma. A person with a long history of smoking should be examined for an intranasal or paranasal sinus epidermoid cancer. All patients must have a laboratory examination. The complete blood cell count evaluates the hematocrit and signs of leukemias. Prothrombin time, partial thromboplastin time, platelet count, and Ivy bleeding time evaluate possible coagulopathies.

The majority of nose bleeds occur anteriorly from the nasal septum and cease spontaneously. If the nose is actively bleeding, the origin can often be seen by visual examination with a head light, nasal speculum, and nasal suction. An actively bleeding nose is treated as follows: A cotton pledget moistened in 4% cocaine is placed against the nasal septum, as it is a good anesthetic for further work and a potent vasoconstrictor. If a definite bleeding site is identified, it may be cauterized with a silver nitrate stick. Cauterization of both sides of the nasal septum should not be done because of the risk of creating a septal perforation. If the bleeding is controlled at this point, it is wise to reduce the air flow through the nose for 5 days by placing a small piece of cotton in the nose. The cotton is saturated with petrolatum or other ointment and it can be changed daily or twice daily by the patient. Recurrent or uncontrollable nose bleeds should be treated by trained personnel, commonly with an anterior nasal pack. Most emergency department physicians are skilled at this, but if not, a head and neck surgeon should be consulted.

Posterior nose bleeds are usually arterial and are often profuse. A head and neck surgeon should be called immediately, and for serious bleeding, 2 to 4 units of blood should be ordered. Posterior nose bleeds are controlled by obstructing the posterior nasal cavity with a Foley balloon or a 4″ × 4″ gauze packing in the nasopharynx. The anterior naris is obstructed with an anterior nasal pack, and the bleeding is tamponaded. This is called an anterior–posterior pack. All patients with posterior nose bleeds are admitted to the hospital and should be under the care of a head and neck surgeon. Figure 3-1 is an algorithm for the diagnosis and treatment of epistaxis.

Some physicians use anterior–posterior packs for 5 days, others for 3 days, and some immediately use arterial ligation. These are options for the patients and the surgeons.

Case Study: Epistaxis

A 42-year-old steel worker presented to the emergency department with a profusely bleeding nose. Pressure to the outside of the nose temporarily stopped the bleeding. The bleeding had begun spontaneously 15 minutes earlier. The patient denied trauma, but had taken two aspirin that morning for a backache. His blood pressure was 160/90. The patient asked for a cigarette, but before he could reach for one, he vomited bright red blood. The nose began bleeding again. Blood was drawn for complete blood cell count, prothrombin time, partial thromboplastin time, platelet count, and typing and cross matching for 4 U. Lactated Ringer's was started using an IV catheter. Bleeding was from the left side of the nose. A No. 18 Foley catheter was passed through the nose, inflated with 20 ml water, and pulled back against the posterior nasal choana. Blood now poured out anteriorly. An anterior nasal pack was inserted using $\frac{1}{2}$-inch plain gauze moistened with povidone-iodine ointment. This controlled the bleeding. Mask oxygen therapy was begun. The patient's blood pressure was 180/95 and the pulse 120. Administration of 25 mg meperidine hydrochloride IV over 2 minutes caused a rapid fall in blood pressure to 110/60 with a pulse of 140. Rapid infusion of 500 ml of Ringer's lactate brought the pressure up to 130/80 with a pulse of 100. The hematocrit was 35, but a repeat hematocrit after the first liter of fluid was given was 25. Two units of blood were given. The patient was admitted to the head and neck surgery service.

The same afternoon a 12-year-old boy entered the emergency

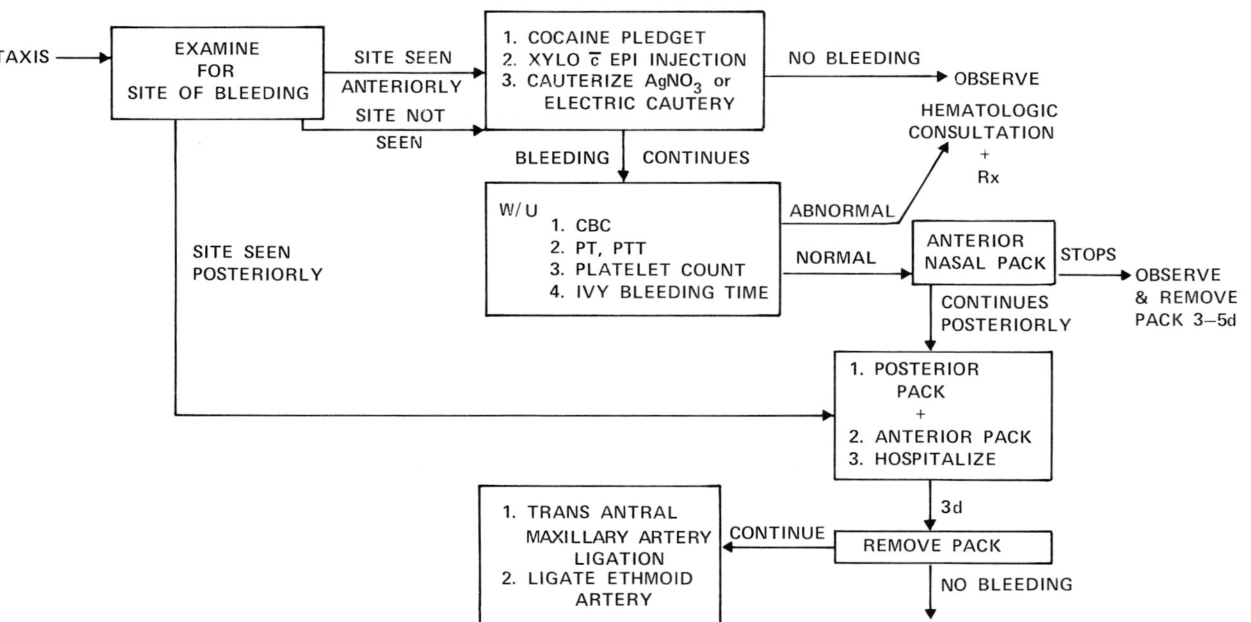

Figure 3.1. Algorithm for evaluation of epistaxis.

61

department soaked with blood. He had been watching television and suddenly began bleeding profusely from the nose. Just as suddenly, the bleeding stopped. History was not helpful, except that the boy's voice had become slightly hyponasal (such as occurs with a stuffy nose) over the past month. Examination was normal except that the soft palate seemed full. A head and neck surgery consultation was requested. Examination of the nasopharynx revealed a large, pulsating mass. A tentative diagnosis of angiofibroma was made, and the patient was admitted to the hospital the following morning for diagnostic angiography.

SINUSITIS

"Sinusitis is this country's most common health care complaint." It affects in excess of 31 million people annually. In 1989, there were almost 16 million physician visits for complaints of sinus disease. Approximately $150 million were spent for cold products prescribed by physicians (from Kennedy, D.W. Otolaryngology—Head and Neck Surgery, 103, #5, Part 2 p 847, 1990).

Rhinitis in the form of an acute upper RTI infection, on the average, afflicts every American twice a year. Virtually everyone suffering from an upper RTI infection initially develops a clear nasal discharge emanating both from the nose and from the paranasal sinuses. This invariably develops into a bacterial superinfection, manifest clinically as a green or yellow mucopurulent nasal discharge. During the upper RTI, many patients have signs and symptoms of paranasal sinus disease and a certain percentage of these develop acute sinusitis. Twenty percent of Americans suffer from one form or another of chronic inflammatory nasal and paranasal sinus disease.

The diagnosis and treatment of sinusitis is currently evolving rapidly, and, hence, no two physicians treat it in the same manner. Two concepts are new; first, plain sinus films have a high false-negative and false-positive incidence, and therefore have been replaced by CT scans. CT scans are expensive, involve 1 to 2 cGY of radiation exposure, and cannot be obtained as quickly or as frequently as conventional plain films. The second development is that there is now a better understanding of the pathophysiology of sinusitis and the ablative morbid sinus procedures have been replaced with new physiologic reconstructive procedures. The major paranasal sinuses, including the frontal sinus, the maxillary sinus, and the majority of the ethmoid sinuses, drain into the middle meatus in and around the anterior ethmoid air cells, an area called the ostiomeatal complex. The anterior ethmoid cells themselves have a poor drainage system, are easily inflamed, and when inflammation occurs, they obstruct maxillary, frontal, and ethmoid sinus ostia, creating stasis and then sinusitis in the maxillary, frontal, and remaining ethmoid sinuses.

The goal of paranasal sinus treatment is to identify the cause of the inflammation, reduce that inflammation, and reestablish drainage from all of the paranasal sinuses. This is done medically with antibiotics and anti-inflammatory medicines. It is performed surgically by endoscopic sinus surgery, an operation that resects the anterior ethmoid sinuses and enlarges the major natural sinus ostia.

To aid in better understanding of evolving treatment, some historical insight is provided. In the 1930s and 1940s, the diagnosis of sinusitis was made clinically. It was often confirmed by eliciting tenderness over the sinus by percussion, and the skilled clinician could transilluminate the maxillary sinus and determine whether it was filled with air or fluid. As antibiotics became available, sinus disease was treated with antibiotics, and when it failed to resolve within a short time, the sinus was irrigated and drained. In the early days, many clinicians were able to cannulate the natural sinus ostia. This required a skill that was lost by most otolaryngologists in the 1950s and 1960s, by which time, the diagnosis of sinusitis was made by history and by radiographic examination. Physical examinations, such as percussion and transillumination, were not deemed to be accurate, and because the radiographs were so readily available, they were used in lieu of transillumination. When the sinusitis failed to respond to antibiotics, its presence was confirmed radiographically and the sinus was drained, most commonly by inserting an 18- or 20-gauge spinal needle into the maxillary sinus. This could be done intranasally through the inferior meatus or transorally through the canine fossa. With the nasal cavity vasoconstricted and a needle in the sinus, water or saline could be irrigated through the maxillary sinus and the gelatinous mucopurulent material of the maxillary sinus flushed out through its natural sinus ostia and, retrieved from a basin. Appropriate cultures were made and with the abscess drained, natural host defenses, aided by antibiotic therapy, would cure the disease. Occasionally, repeated irrigations were required and if this failed, surgical exploration and drainage were recommended. The surgery for the maxillary sinus involved making a window between the maxillary sinus and the nose, the so-called naso-antral window. This was most commonly created in the inferior meatus. It was created either intranasally, or by Caldwell–Luc operation, thereby gaining access to the sinus underneath the upper lip and through the anterior face of the maxilla. Under direct vision, a large naso-antral window was then created. The ethmoid sinuses were treated simply by eradication, performed intranasally through a Caldwell–Luc procedure, (transantral ethmoidectomy), or externally through an incision made between the nose and the medial canthus. Frontal sinusitis was approached directly either through an incision along the brow or occasionally, particularly in women, via a coronal incision. The skin of the forehead was reflected forward, and the frontal sinus opened through the frontal bone.

Fortunately, sphenoid sinusitis was uncommon, but when it existed, it was approached in much the same fashion as ethmoid sinusitis.

There were two problems with the above approach. First, the surgery itself was terribly uncomfortable and was corrective only sometimes. Second, it caused a moderate amount of morbidity and, so, even if the patient survived the surgery and the primary sinus disease was cured, there were intrasinus scar tissue, crusting, infection, and congestion; sinus discomfort became a part of life.

The development of rigid nasal endoscopes permitted direct examination of the natural sinus ostia. With the advent of CT scans, the inaccuracies of conventional radiography became grossly apparent; with the recognition of normal paranasal sinus drainage avenues, endoscopic sinus surgery was developed and the entire approach to paranasal sinus disease began to change. It continues to evolve, and time will tell which tests, approaches, and procedures will be most widely adopted. In all probability, the primary care physicians, because of their skills, the equipment available to them, and the type of patients they see, will have one approach to sinus disease, and the otolaryngologist, who has a referral sinus practice, will diagnose and treat in a different fashion.

Case Study: Sinusitis

A 26-year-old college student presented with left facial pain. She had had a cold that persisted for 10 days. One day before examination, she began to notice pain and pressure over her left cheek. She went to her dentist who took an X ray and told her she had a sinus infection. He referred her for treatment. History was unremarkable. The patient's temperature was 101°F. The nose was clear, but mucopurulent material was dripping from the nasopharynx. Percussion over the left maxillary sinus elicited tenderness. The patient had a classic left maxillary sinusitis. This was treated with penicillin and a saline nasal douche. The patient was instructed to return if her symptoms did not disappear in 3 to 4 days or if they recurred.

Most can agree on the evaluation and treatment of acute maxillary sinusitis. Typically, this is found in an individual who suffers an upper RTI and, as a part of that viral illness, develops a superimposed bacterial rhinitis, presenting as a purulent rhinorrhea. The sinus ostia become inflamed and are eventually occluded. Trapped secretions become infected and, typically, at the time the cold should have cleared, the patient notices pain and pressure over one or the other maxillary sinuses. There may or may not be involvement of the ethmoids or of the frontals, but certainly their involvement is less commonly evident.

These patients will present with pain and pressure over one or both maxillary sinuses. They often feel sick and may have an elevated temperature. Most have a purulent postnasal discharge, but a few have a purulent anterior nasal discharge. Conventional anterior rhinoscopy with a flashlight or even a nasal speculum will reveal little. Rigid endoscopy of the middle meatus will identify mucopurulent material emanating from the natural sinus ostia. Examination of the posterior oropharynx may reveal mucopurulent material coursing down the posterior or lateral oropharyngeal wall. Sometimes this discharge is absent, but red streaks or inflamed mucosa may be evident. Cervical adenopathy is not an early sign in adults nor is it a particularly useful or diagnostic sign in children. Percussion directly over the sinus will often elicit pain of that sinus. If it is a maxillary sinus, that same type of pain can be induced by tapping on the canine or molar teeth.

The diagnosis of sinusitis is made entirely on the clinical presentation. Table 3.1 lists the normal pathogens isolated from acute sinusitis. Treatment is a prescription for 7 to 10 days of antibiotics. Penicillin is excellent for its streptococci and anaerobic coverage, but lacks coverage for resistent species of *H. influenza*. Amoxicillin may be a better drug for this reason. Erythromycin remains the drug of choice for those who are penicillin sensitive. Cephalosporins, trimethoprimsulfa, ampicillin with clavulonic acid, and other broad-spectrum, more expensive, antibiotics are all second-line drugs.

The patient can improve nasal hygiene by sniffing 2 or 3 drops of

Table 3.1 Organisms from Maxillary Sinus Disease*

Streptococcus pneumoniae
Hemophilus influenzae
Viruses
Moraxella catarrhalis
Group A *Streptococcus*
Staphylococcus aureus
Gram-negative bacilli
    Proteus
    Klebsiella
    Escherichia coli
Pseudomonas aeruginosa
Anaerobes
    Peptostreptococcus
    Bacteroides

*The organisms at the top of the list are most common in acute paranasal sinus disease, those at the bottom are more common in chronic paranasal sinus disease

saline and then blowing this back out. The saline douche can be made at home or obtained as a prescription item. Antihistamine decongestants have not proved useful, because histamine is not active in bacterial rhinosinusitis. Oral decongestants such as ephedrine can be used for symptomatic relief. Antihistamines and antihistamine decongestant combinations have the potential disadvantage of making the secretions thicker and of reducing ciliary function, thereby decreasing the clearance of purulent sinus fluids.

Topical decongestants such as phenylephrine and oxymetazoline (Afrin®) decongest the nose and theoretically facilitate drainage through the natural sinus ostia. Unfortunately, many individuals who acquire sinusitis already have a compromised nasal passage, and even though they are warned about using the nasal sprays sparingly for 2 or 3 days, they continue to use them for a longer period and become nasal addicts; a condition called rhinitis medica mentosa.

Therefore, a normal prescription is for Pen VK® 250 mg, four times daily for 10 days, or for amoxicillin 250 mg three times a day for 10 days. A prescription for a decongestant such as pseudoephedrine can be given if there is excessive nasal congestion and discomfort. The patient is advised to use it sparingly. The patient is instructed to use saline nose drops four times a day. Steam inhalation for 5 to 10 minutes helps loosen secretions. Once the gelatinous secretions that have collected in the sinus are blown out, the sinuses begin to drain normally, the infection resolves, the pain and pressure dissipate, and the patient rapidly recovers.

For those individuals who feel they require analgesics, acetaminophen is the drug of choice, followed by aspirin, and acetaminophen or aspirin with codeine, respectively.

Those individuals who do not improve will normally return 2 to 4 days after the initial visit. Presumably, they have an ostial obstruction that is not allowing drainage and may have bacteria resistant to the prescribed drugs. At this point, some physicians would obtain a sinus X ray; however, such X rays have a high degree of inaccuracy. Assuming it is the maxillary sinus that is involved, most otolaryngologists irrigate the sinus. This is most commonly done by vasoconstricting the middle meatus by spraying the nasal cavity with 0.5% phenylephrine. An 18- or 20-gauge spinal needle is then twisted through the maxillary bone into the maxillary sinus. This can be done intranasally through the inferior meatus or under the upper lip through the canine fossa. In either case, 1% lidocaine with 1:100,000 epinephrine is injected. The spinal needle is placed through the mucosa and up against the bone and then with a twisting or drilling motion drilled through the bone and into the sinus. The patient is instructed to lean forward and 20 cc to 50 cc of sterile irrigant is flushed through the sinus. There is often resistance at first and then a 5- or 6-cc viscous fluid exudes from the sinus. If the patient is leaning forward, this will flow out through the nose and can be caught in a sterile basin. The material can be sent for culture and sensitivity. It is probably the irrigation that affects the cure, but many practitioners will also choose to change the antibiotic. Some do so empirically, some wait for culture and sensitivity results.

Case Study: Acute Maxillary Sinusitis

A case example will help accentuate several points. An 18-year-old secretary came to my office with a history of a cold 1 week previously. Just as the cold seemed to be abating, she developed pain on the left side of her face. She saw her dentist, who referred her to me. Examination of the nose was normal, the oropharynx revealed a mucopurulent postnasal discharge. Her temperature was 101°F orally. Finger percussion over the left maxilla elicited pain. A clinical diagnosis of acute maxillary sinusitis was made. The patient was given prescriptions for amoxicillin 250 mg po three times a day for 10 days and advised to use Sudafed® for nasal stuffiness. The patient was also told to mix 1 teaspoon of salt in a glass of water and to put two drops of this solution into each nostril four times a day. She was to sniff this in and then blow it out. She was instructed not to return if the symptoms abated. However, if the symptoms persisted, recurred, or increased she should return immediately.

The patient returned 2 weeks later stating that the symptoms had disappeared on the antibiotic therapy but as soon as she stopped taking the amoxicillin the symptoms returned. The examination showed the same results. This is an older case, and at this time plain sinus X rays were used to evaluate and diagnose inflammatory sinus illness. Figure 3.2 shows skull positioning for the four standard sinus X rays. Figure 3.3 shows a normal sinus series.

The patient's Waters' view (Figure 3.4) showed an air-fluid level on the left side and an opacified sinus on the right side. To document this as an air-fluid level the patient's head was tilted slightly to the right, and the repeat Waters view showed a shift in the air-fluid level. Sinus irrigation was recommended. The nose was vasoconstricted, and on each side the mucosa in the canine fossa was anesthetized and a 20-gauge spinal needle inserted into the maxillary sinus. The irrigated pus was collected and sent for culture and sensitivity. The patient was placed on amoxicillin with clavulonic acid. For the first 48 hours, 500 mg was prescribed every 8 hours. For the ensuing 12 days, 250 mg was prescribed every 8 hours. The symptoms did not recur.

If one or two irrigations had failed to clear the infection, a nasal work-up would have been initiated and, based on the findings of that work-up, appropriate therapy recommended.

As has been stated, plain sinus radiographs are no longer used to evaluate acute sinus disease, and when, in fact, a radio-

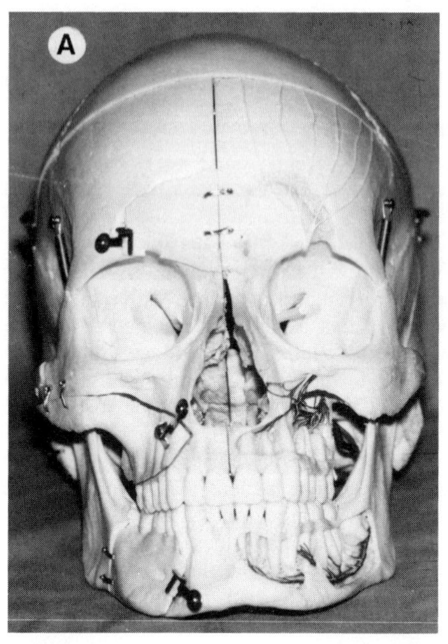

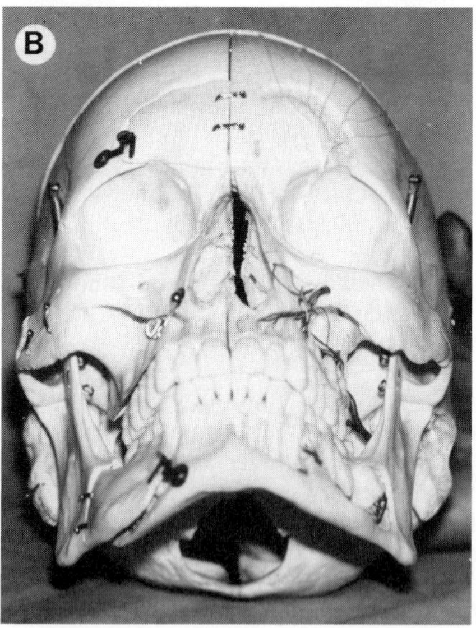

Figure 3.2. Views of the skull showing position of the head for each of the four standard sinus X rays, assuming that the X ray beam is horizontal. (A) Posteroanterior view. (B) Waters' view. *(Continued on p. 69.)*

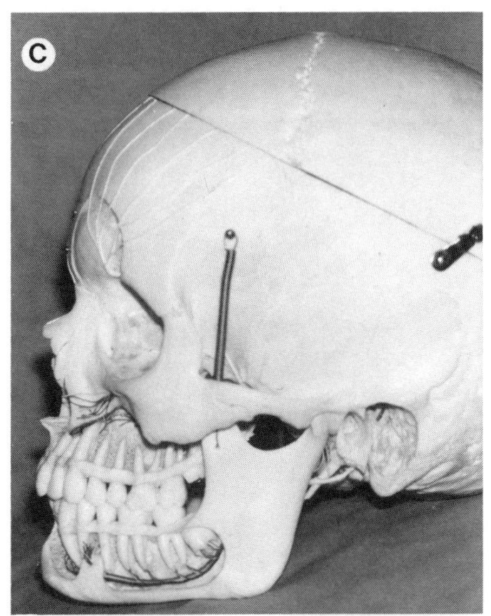

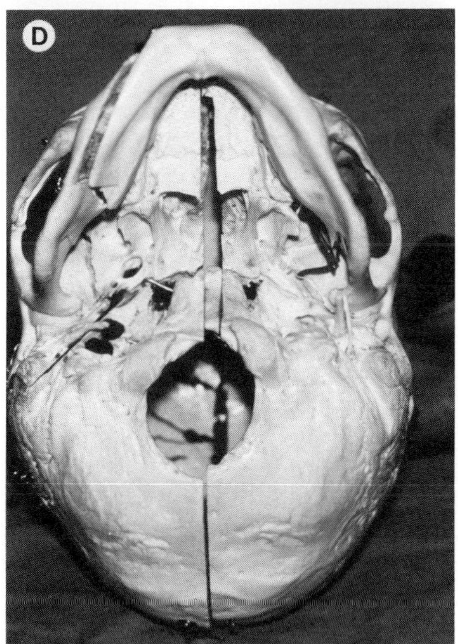

Figure 3.2. **(continued)** (C) Lateral view. (D) Submental vertical view.

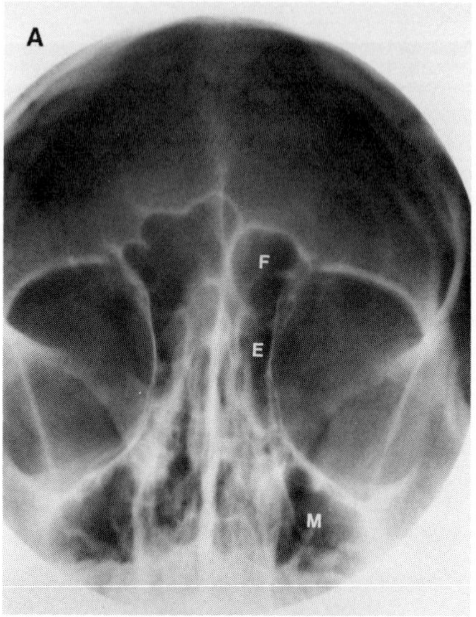

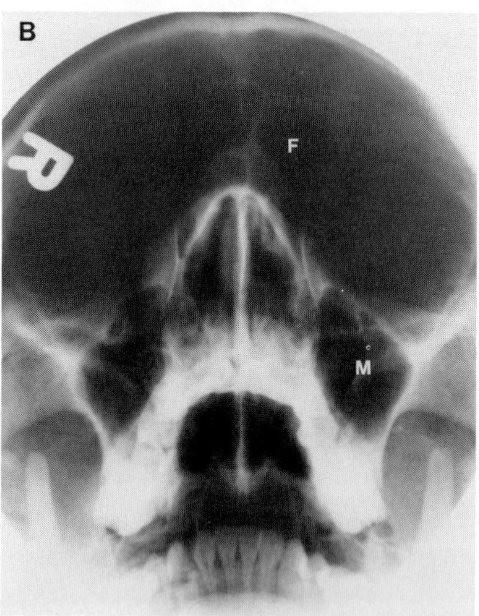

Figure 3.3.   Normal results of sinuses series of X rays. Sinus films are taken with the patient upright, in a coned-down focus, and with soft-tissue penetration. (A) Posteroanterior view. (B) Waters' view. *(Continued on p. 71.)*

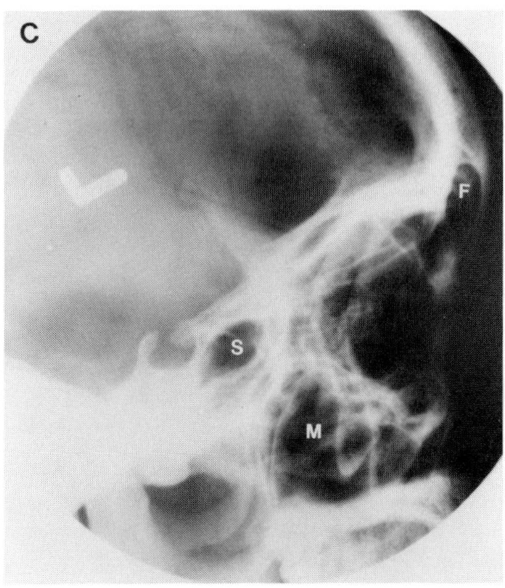

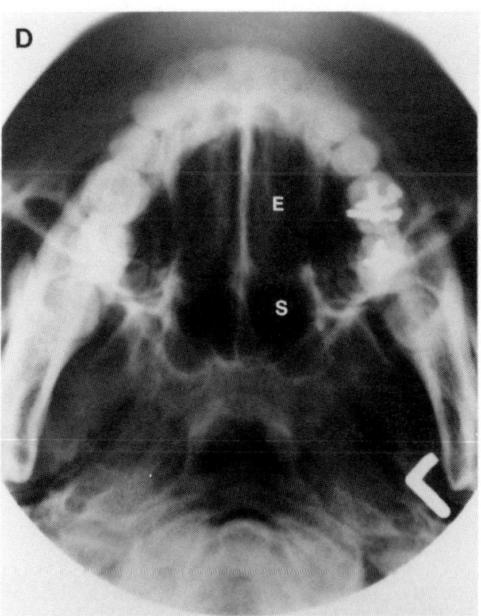

Figure 3.3. (continued) (C) Lateral view. (D) SMV view. F = frontal sinus, E = ethmoid sinus, M = maxillary sinus, S = sphenoid sinus.

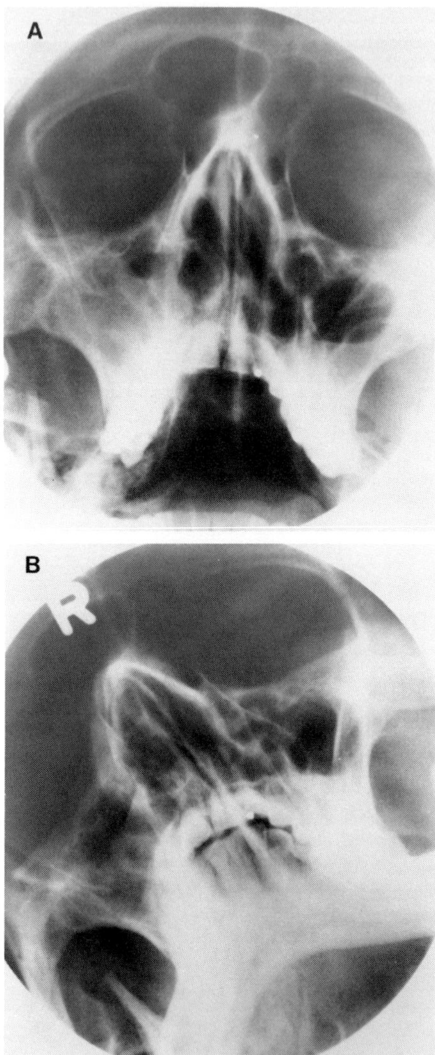

Figure 3.4.   X rays of acute maxillary sinusitis. (A) Waters' view showing an air-fluid level in the left maxillary sinus and opacification of the right maxillary sinus. Note the small air bubble in the superior medial corner of this sinus. (B) Waters' view with the head tilted to the right. Note how the air-fluid level orientation changes in the left maxillary sinus. *(Continued on p. 72.)*

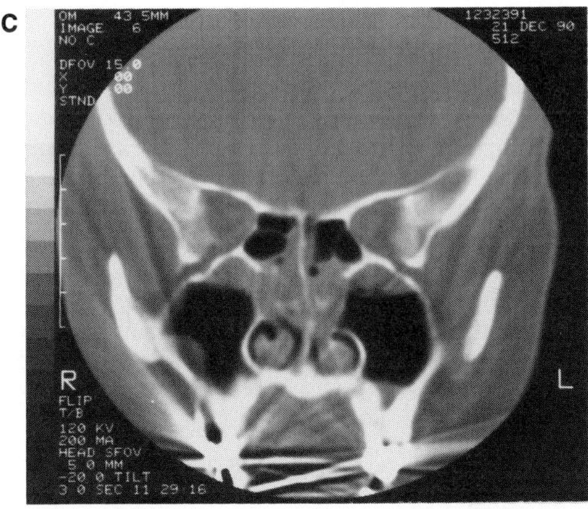

Figure 3.4. **(continued)** (C) Coronal CT on an individual with symptoms of acute maxillary sinusitis. Note the extensive anterior ethmoidal disease obstructing the ostial meatal complex and the accumulation of fluid in both maxillary sinuses.

graph is indicated, sinus CTs are ordered. Figure 3.4C is a coronal CT that demonstrates the kind of findings that might commonly be observed in an individual with acute maxillary sinusitis. Note that the primary disease is in the anterior ethmoids in the area called the ostiomeatal complex. It is because of the disease in this region that the natural sinus ostia for the maxillary sinuses are obstructed and, therefore, fluid and infection has accumulated in the maxillary sinus. Because the patient is positioned upside down, air-fluid levels are now seen at the top of the sinuses.

It is interesting that European physicians approach this slightly differently. When the patient fails to improve, they will perform a maxillary sinus endoscopy, typically through the canine fossa. This involves inserting a 5-mm diameter trochar through the face of the maxilla. This is not a major procedure, but by the same token, is more involved than simply inserting an 18- or 20-gauge needle. With the trochar into the maxillary sinus, a sterile aspirate and culture are obtained. The sinus can be irrigated directly and the sinus examined endoscopically for tumors, polyps, ostial obstruction, and so forth.

Some American otolaryngologists will irrigate two or three times, some will perform maxillary sinus endoscopy earlier and, in some cases with either procedure, the acute sinus disease is cleared. An algorithm for the evaluation and treatment of sinus infection is shown in Figure 3.5.

Sometimes the disease is not cleared; it becomes indolent and presents as chronic sinusitis. Chronic sinusitis includes that disease that has been refractory to prior treatments and disease that has been indolent and has slowly become an increasing problem.

These individuals require a more complex and thorough work-up. The nature and degree of this work-up differs among both physicians and institutions. Table 3.2 lists those tests that are performed at the UCSD Nasal Dysfunction Clinic.

A history is appropriate. The physical examination should include endoscopic rhinoscopy. Rigid endoscopy is preferable to flexible rhi-

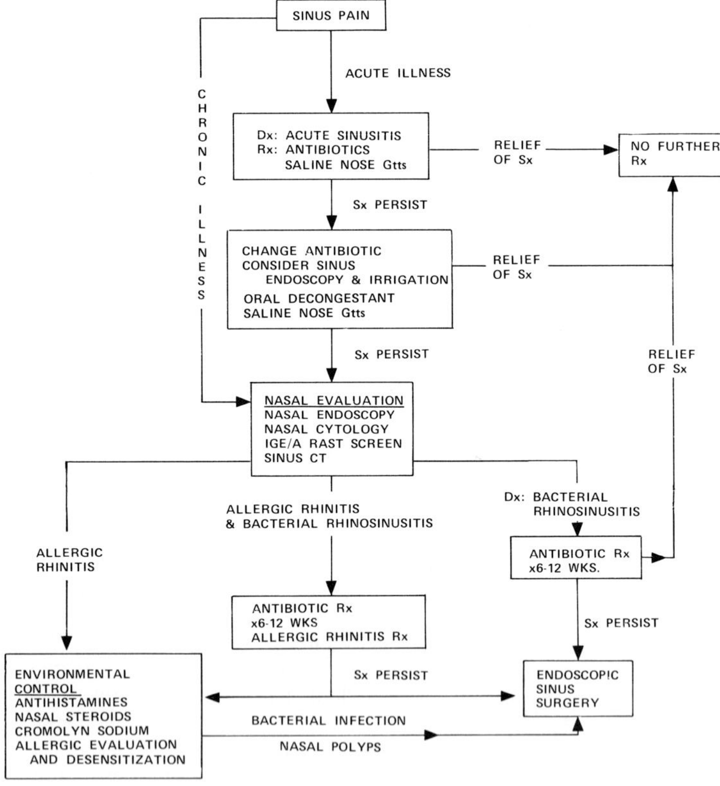

Figure 3.5.   Algorithm for the evaluation and treatment of sinusitis.

Table 3.2 Evaluation for Nasal Dysfunction

History
Anterior rhinoscopy
Oropharyngeal examination
Nasal endoscopy
Olfactory testing
Rhinomanometry
Nasal cytology
IgE level
RAST inhalant panel screen
Sinus CT

---

noscopy. The oropharynx should be examined. Important findings in the nose are patency of the airway and presence or absence of a septal deviation, particularly one that is obstructive. The mucosa of the inferior turbinate is reflective of the mucosa of the remainder of the nasal cavity. If this is inflamed, it implies a bacterial infection; if it is edematous and either pale or bluish in color, this is most consistent with an allergic problem. The presence of blood or of a tumor is a significant finding, as is presence of polyps. The presence of secretions is also a pertinent finding. Clear or white secretions are found in allergic rhinitis. Purulent secretions are found in bacterial rhinitis.

Case Study: Pansinusitis and Asthma

A 49-year-old woman enjoyed excellent health throughout her childhood and early adult life. Approximately 1 year ago she developed asthmatic symptoms and initiated therapy. Four months ago the asthma worsened and she required hospitalization for systemic steroids and bronchodilators. Around this time she noted difficulty with nasal breathing that progressed to symptoms of sinus disease including pain and pressure over the sinuses and finally a purulent postnasal discharge. The symptoms progressed to the point where she was unable to breathe through her nose. Medications included doxycycline, astemizole, Actifed®, theophylline, albuterol, impratropium bromide, Afrin®, intranasal steroids, and cromolyn sodium. She had no known medical allergies.

Anterior rhinoscopy revealed the nose totally obstructed by polypoid tissue. Endoscopy was not possible. The oropharynx showed an edematous mucosa consistent with an allergic disease. Rhinomanometry was attempted. No measurable airflow was possible prior to decongestants. Following decongestant spray, resistances in the right and left nostril, respectively, were 4.2 cm and 4.7 cm of $H_2O/L/sec$. These are normal. The nasal cytogram revealed numerous eosinophils with basophilic cells and neutrophils. Few bacteria were present. The IgE was 180 U/mL with the upper limits of normal being 40 U/mL. The RAST inhalant panel revealed no sensitivities to grasses, trees, animal danders, mites, or fungi. The CT scan shown in Figure 3.6 demonstrated diffuse mucoperiosteal thickening involving the sphenoid sinuses, the ethmoid sinuses, and the maxillary sinuses. Diffuse mucus membrane thickening was seen in the nasal cavity.

Surgery was recommended and accepted. A septoplasty was performed, in part to improve the anatomic airway and in part to improve endoscopic access to the ethmoid sinuses. Endoscopic sinus surgery was performed. Both an anterior and a posterior ethmoidectomy were performed. The natural maxillary sinus ostia were enlarged. The frontal recess cells were resected, and drainage was established to the frontal sinuses. The sphenoid sinus ostia were identified and opened, thereby draining the sphenoid sinuses into the posterior naval cavity. All the nasal polyps were resected.

Postoperatively, the patient made an uneventful recovery. The nasal packing was removed on postoperative day 3. Nasal irrigations using a Water Pic® with an Ethicore nasal adaptor were initiated on postoperative day 10, and the patient began nasal medications, including nasal steroids and cromolyn sodium, 3 weeks following surgery.

Immediately following surgery the patient's lungs made a dramatic improvement, and within 1 or 2 weeks she could tell that her nose and paranasal sinuses felt dramatically better. She had an overall sense of once again being healthy.

Not all asthmatics have sinus disease, and not all asthmatics with sinus disease require endoscopic sinus surgery. However, some asthmatics clearly deteriorate when their nasal and paranasal sinus disease exacerbates, as typified by the above individual who made dramatic pulmonary improvement with appropriate management of her sinus disease.

Rhinoscopy should examine the entire nasal cavity, with particular attention to the middle meatus. Purulent secretions emanating from the middle meatus or from the sinus ostia indicate a bacterial sinus infection.

The oropharynx is a good indicator of nasal pathology. The majority of nasal secretions are transported posteriorly and flow down the posterior and lateral oropharyngeal walls. In allergic conditions, the mucosa will be pale and edematous. In bacterial conditions, the mucosa will appear red and inflamed. Clear secretions indicate an allergic or vasomotor condition; purulent secretions indicate a bacterial condition.

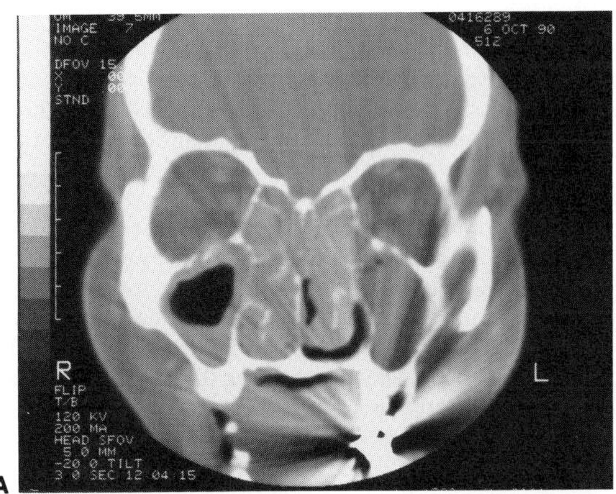

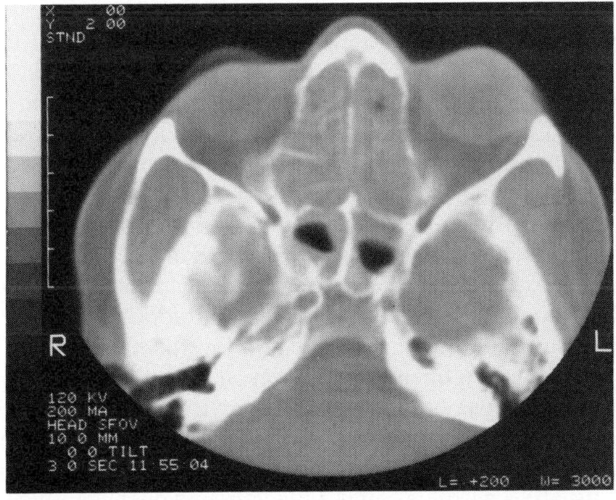

Figure 3.6. (A) Coronal computed tomography (CT) scan demonstrating extensive nasal and paranasal sinus disease. The ethmoid sinuses are completely filled with inflammatory tissue. One cannot differentiate fluid from soft tissue. The olfactory cleft is obstructed. The left maxillary sinus appears to be filled with fluid or soft tissue swelling. The right maxillary sinus shows extensive mucosal swelling. The nasal cavity is also filled with swollen, inflammed tissue. At this particular time, the right nasal cavity appears worse than the left. However, both are severely diseased. (B) Axial CT scan demonstrating extensive ethmoidal disease involving both the anterior and posterior ethmoid sinuses. Mucosal swelling is seen in the sphenoid sinuses.

Although the remainder of the head and neck examination is important for all patients presenting to an otolaryngologist, it does relatively little to better define the nasal condition.

Laboratory data are also needed. Laboratory investigation should include cytologic examination of the mucous of the inferior turbinate (nasal cytology) and rhinomanometry to look at the nasal airflow and the change of airflow in response to a topical spray.

Blood is drawn for an IgE level and a RAST screen for 10 common inhalant allergens. A sinus CT is ordered. Based on the history, the examination, and the results of the laboratory tests, further information may be required. Serum immunoglobulins may be useful when looking for IgA deficiency or IgG subclass deficiencies. For those who are allergic, a full RAST panel may better define the individual's allergies. Other tests may be ordered as circumstances dictate.

Case Study: Revision Sinus Surgery

The patient was a 32-year-old software engineer with a long history of sinusitis, difficulty breathing through his nose, nasal polyps, and asthma. His asthma was, to a large degree, affected by the condition of his paranasal sinuses, and hence 3 years previously, he underwent exterpative sinus surgery including a Caldwell–Luc and antral windows. He also had bilateral intranasal ethmoidectomies. In the early postoperative period, he felt better, feeling that both his allergies and his asthma were symptomatically improved. However, over the course of several years, the asthmatic symptoms worsened and his exercise tolerance decreased. He had also had recurrent episodes of sinusitis and had required repeated, prolonged antibiotic therapy.

He was referred to the UCSD Nasal Dysfunction Clinic. The only additional pertinent history was an awareness of a diminution in his sense of smell 5 years previously, with a marked increase in this loss immediately following the previous ethmoid surgery. He had no parosmia, but had had occasional phantosmias, usually a gasoline smell. Olfactory and odor-identification testing indicated mild hyposmia in the left nostril and anosmia or severe hyposmia in the right nostril. Rhinomanometry before and after phenylephrine showed a nasal airway resistance in the right nostril to be 5.4 cm and 4.2 cm H_2O/L/sec. and in the left nostril 4.7 and 3.8, respectively. The right nostril, therefore, showed some increased airway resistance prior to decongestant. Both airways were reasonably patent after decongestants. The nasal cytogram revealed significant numbers of eosinophils and a few basophilic cells. There was no evidence of infection. An IgE was 40 U/mL, which is at the upper limits of normal. The RAST inhalant screen was negative. Nasal endoscopy revealed a posterior septal deflection and an ostiomeatal complex filled with mucopus and inflammatory tissue. The nose was clearly malodorous, and the middle turbinates were strikingly absent, a consequence of the previous intranasal ethmoidectomy. The CT scan is shown in Figure 3.7.

Septoplasty and endoscopic sinus surgery were performed. At the time of surgery, the nasal cavity was filled with muco-purulent polypoid material. This material was carefully re-moved. Additional ethmoid sinuses were opened and drainage facilitated. The natural middle meatal maxillary sinus ostia were large, however, obstructed by polypoid tissue. This polypoid tissue was resected. The agger nasi cells surrounding the frontal sinus drainage contained mucopurulent material. These cells were resected, and the frontal sinus drainage reestablished.

The patient's postoperative recovery was uneventful. The nasal packing was removed after 3 days. Nasal irrigations with a Water-pik® and an Ethicore® nasal adaptor were initiated on postoperative day 10. The patient was maintained on his asth-matic medicines throughout surgery and the postoperative pe-riod and was begun on intranasal steroids 3 weeks postopera-tively.

His sense of smell has not returned substantially, probably because the olfactory epithelium was inadvertently destroyed at the previous sinus surgery. His asthma and exercise tolerance have improved dramatically. His nose has remained clean and he has felt well.

The differential diagnosis for nasal and paranasal sinus disease is lengthy, but by far the most common diagnoses fall under three head-ings. Tumors are perhaps the least common, but certainly of the most concern. They include a variety of malignancies, such as epidermoid carcinoma, and a variety of benign tumors, such as papilloma. The nasal endoscopy and the CT scan followed by a biopsy should identify and diagnose the condition.

Case Study: Vasomotor Rhinitis

Mr. X was a 45-year-old man referred for evaluation of sinus headaches. He had been to many physicians, none of whom had been able to help and, hence, was referred to the UNDC. The history was that of episodic facial and forehead pain. This usually began in the afternoon and normally would persist into the evening in spite of analgesics or antihistamines. It often had a profuse, watery, nasal discharge associated with the pain and it totally incapacitated his ability to function at work. The entire head and neck examination at this time was normal. A complete

   CLINICAL MANUAL OF OTOLARYNGOLOGY

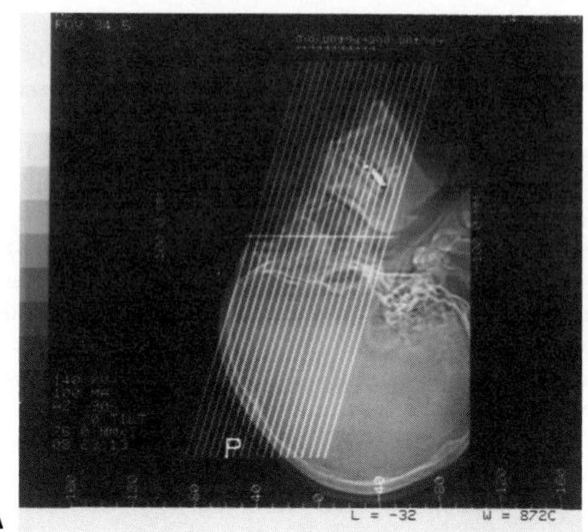

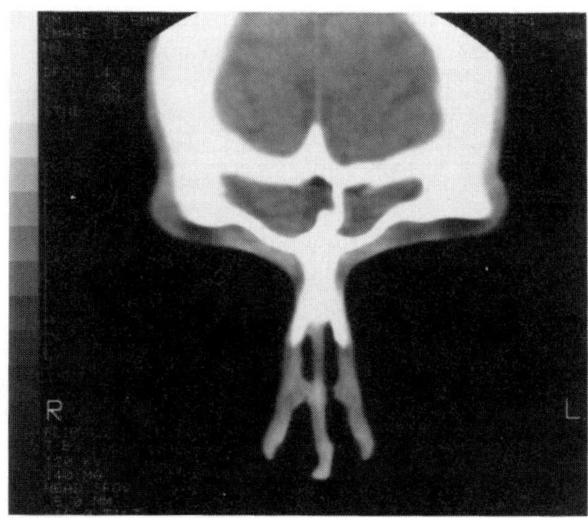

Figure 3.7.   (A) Port film showing the coronal view. (B) Anterior most coronal computed tomography (CT) scan showing both frontal sinuses opacified. See if you can identify which cut this is on the port film. *(Continued on p. 81.)*

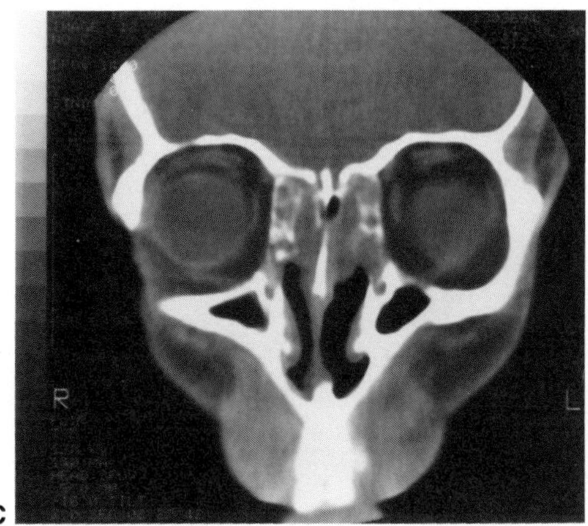

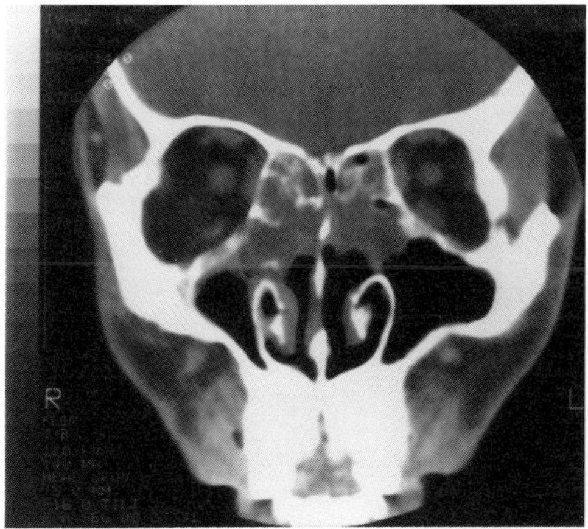

Figure 3.7. (continued) (C) This is the 8th coronal CT scan. Note the eyes and the extraocular muscles contained within the bony orbit. The most anterior portion of the maxillary sinuses are shown. The inferior turbinates are not yet visible. High in the nasal cavity extensive ethmoidal disease is evident. The superior nasal cavity is completely filled with inflammatory tissue. (D) This is the 10th coronal CT. Inferior turbinates are now well seen. Maxillary sinuses are well seen and in these views have little disease. The ethmoid sinuses are totally opacified. A few pockets of air are identified on the left. The polypoid material filling the nasal cavity is evident. *(Continued on p. 82.)*

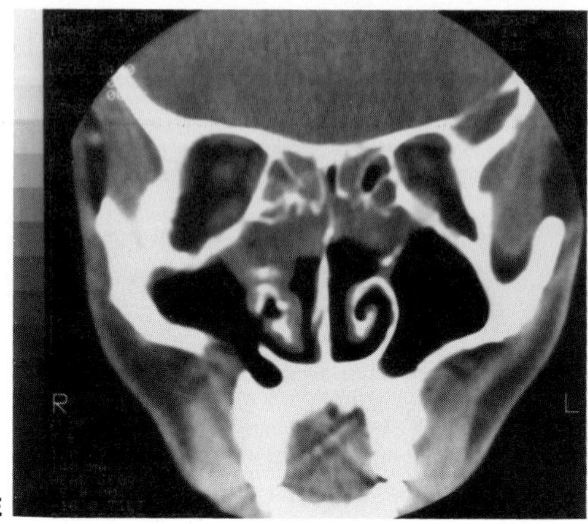

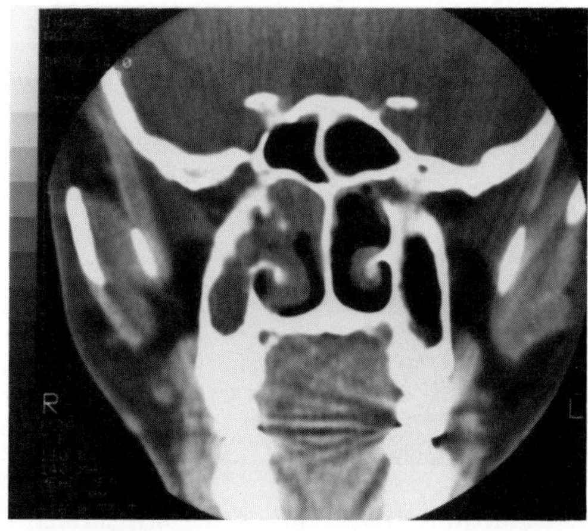

Figure 3.7. (continued) (E) This is the 11th coronal CT. The inferior meatal antrostomy on the right is now evident. The ethmoid disease is obvious and the complete obstruction of the natural maxillary sinus ostia is evident on this and the preceding CT scan. Note the striking absence of the middle turbinates. (F) This is the 14th coronal CT. This shows the most posterior portions of the maxillary sinuses. Posterior ethmoid and posterior maxillary sinus disease is evident on the right. The sphenoid sinuses are seen and are disease free. *(Continued on p. 83.)*

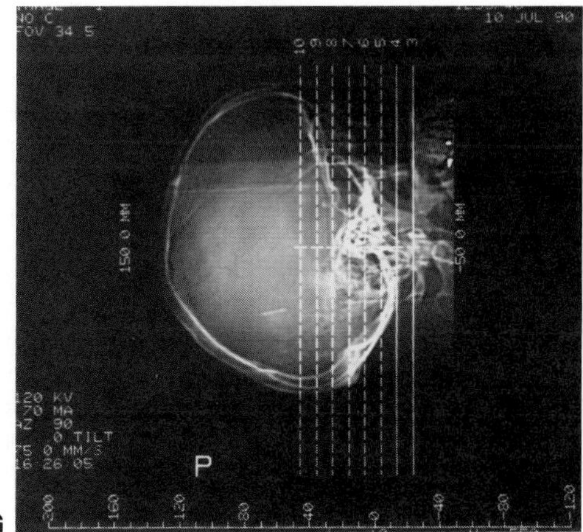

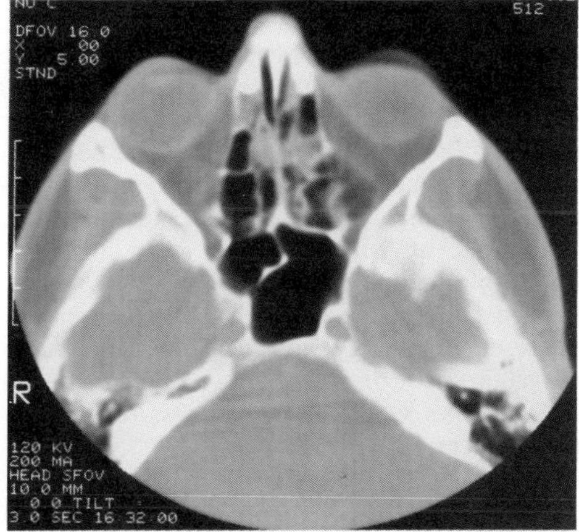

Figure 3.7. **(continued)** (G) This is the axial CT port film. (H) Fifth axial CT scan through the mid-ethmoids showing disease of the ostiomeatal complex.

nasal dysfunction work-up was ordered. The nasal physiology, the sinus CT, the IgE, and the RAST screens all were normal. It was suggested that this was a vasomotor rhinitis, which was a true psychosomatic disorder and one that needed to be dealt with psychiatrically. We explored some of the stresses in his life. I referred him to a psychiatrist. During counseling, it was revealed that he was the child of alcoholic parents and suffered from all the problems associated therewith. He became involved in some short-term counseling and also became involved in a group of adult children of alcoholic parents.

He quickly gave up the nasal steroids and decongestants that I had recommended. I didn't see him in follow-up for 3 months. He had pursued the counseling and group therapy actively and stated that he was truly a new man. He was now sleeping at night, he was happy at home, and was both happy and productive at work.

Stress is a common problem presenting as nasal disease. Vasomotor rhinitis is a psychosomatic disease. It is parasympathetic mediated, as are peptic ulcer disease and functional bowel syndrome. In response to stress, the parasympathetic system is stimulated. The identified target organ is the nasal and paranasal sinus mucosa. The mucosa swells and secretions are induced. The nose becomes congested and anterior or posterior rhinorrhea may be evident. Nasal endoscopy is normal, the IgE and RAST are normal, and the CT scan is normal.

History confirms stress in the patient's life either at home or at work. Typically, the sinus problems come on for a short period. For some individuals, they may begin in the afternoon; for other individuals, they may wake up with them; for some, they are weekend problems similar to migraine headaches.

Antihistamine decongestants, decongestants alone, or nasal steroids may lessen the symptomatology; however, optimal therapy is to identify this as a psychosomatic disorder, appropriately instruct the patient, and have him or her seek help either in stress reduction or in more aggressive psychotherapy.

Case Study: Allergic Rhinitis

A 30-year-old nurse complained that she couldn't breathe through her nose. This was readily evident for she was an obligate mouth breather. The history was classic for allergic rhinitis because the problem was worse in the spring and the fall. Her nose itched, as did her eyes. There was no infectious component and both sides of her nose seemed to be equally involved. Nasal examination revealed a swollen, bluish mucosa, almost totally occluding the airway. The posterior oropharynx was pale and edematous. A nasal cytology was loaded with the eosinophils and the basophils. The serum IgE was markedly elevated, and the RAST screen showed mild allergy to molds and grasses and a very strong reaction to cat epithelium. However, the woman would not consider giving up her cat. Nasal steroids were prescribed and she was advised to do whatever she could to reduce the allergic load in the environment.

For follow-up visit 6 weeks later, she had made some improvement on nasal steroids and environmental control. The cat remained in the house and her nose, for the most part, remained extremely stuffy. Again it was affirmed that if she really wished to be better, she would need to get rid of the cat. She reaffirmed that this was not going to occur.

She returned once again, 3 months later. At first glance she was still an obligate mouth breather, and the allergic rhinitis persisted. She then related that her 16-month-old daughter had developed asthma, and her pediatrician had now advised her that she had to get rid of the cat. In the interest of both daughter and patient this was done. The daughter's asthma improved, the patient's allergic rhinitis diminished and my son and I have a beautiful Persian cat.

The most common nasal disorders are inflammatory in origin. They may be allergic, bacterial, or, often, a mixture of allergy and infection. The pure allergic disease presents with congestion and a clear or white nasal discharge. The condition may be seasonal or perennial. Endoscopy reveals a swollen pale or blue mucosa. Nasal polyps may be seen emanating from the middle meatus. The oropharynx is pale and edematous, and clear or white secretions may be seen flowing down the pharyngeal walls. Nasal cytology typically, but not necessarily, shows basophils or eosinophils. There may or may not be an obstructive septal component, but typically, airway resistance diminishes (airflow improves) after the mucosa is vasoconstricted with phenylephrine. In IgE-mediated allergy, the serum IgE will be elevated and often specific allergens will be identified on the RAST panel. Classically, the CT scan will be normal; however, if polyps have developed, these will be present in the nasal cavity and may also be found filling the ethmoid sinuses, the maxillary sinuses, and less commonly, the frontal sinuses. In addition, if the polyps are obstructing the sinus ostia, a bacterial infection with opacification may be evident in any or all of the paranasal sinuses.

Treatment involves any or all of the following approaches. First and foremost is environmental control. If specific allergens such as pets are present in the house, they should be removed, but in addition, almost everyone with an allergic diathesis has sensitivity to molds, fungi, mites, dust, and so forth, and to whatever degree the home and work environment can have their allergic load reduced, the patient will do better.

The simplest medical treatment is with antihistamines; certainly the cheapest and simplest therapy would be an over-the-counter nonspecific antihistamine decongestant. Each patient and each physician have their favorites. Examples of such medications include: Actifed®, Ornade®, Drixoral®, Entex®. Although there are five different classes of antihistamines, patient tolerance and patient response is unpredictable. Most individuals should try two or three different medications to determine efficacy and side effects.

Two H1-specific antihistamines available today are terfenadine and astemizole. Terfenadine can be taken on an as needed basis and typically is administered at 1 dose twice a day. Astemizole is taken once a day.

The next medicines to consider are nasal inhalants. Cromolyn sodium blocks mast cells and so, particularly in those individuals with a nasal secretory basophilia, cromolyn sodium (NasalCrom®) delivered one sniff in each nostril four times a day on a prn basis may be efficacious.

The most powerful allergic nasal medications available today are the nasal steroids. Eighty μg (two puffs) is typically instilled in each nostril two or three times daily. Nasal steroids are most efficacious with allergic rhinitis, and have been of some benefit in vasomotor rhinitis. They must be taken on a regular basis because they have a long half-life. Patients using nasal steroids must be careful to discontinue them during periods of bacterial infection, because host resistance to bacterial infection is reduced. When individuals develop an upper respiratory tract infection, the nasal steroids should be discontinued. For those who have a bacterial component to their allergy, protection with an oral antibiotic is strongly advised. If none of the aforementioned regimens are efficacious, referral to an allergist is appropriate. There are two groups who practice in allergy control: otolaryngologists and medical immunologists. In both cases, specific sensitivities are determined and the patient is administered measured doses of the respective allergens in an effort to desensitize to the particular allergen. In some individuals this is effective, and in others the efficacy is uncertain. In any case, desensitization requires intradermal injections that are typically administered three times a week.

There is no surgical therapy for allergy, but those individuals with compounding problems such as a deviated nasal septum or bacterial sinusitis may be advised to consider surgical correction of those problems.

Another cause of inflammatory nasal and paranasal sinus disease is a chronic bacterial infection. Typically, these individuals have been on and off antibiotics. They are better while on the antibiotics and inevitably relapse sometime after discontinuing them.

On examination, the nasal mucosa is inflamed and examination of the middle meatus reveals purulent discharge. The oropharynx has a purulent postnasal drip or evidence thereof. Typically, there is red streaking or red lymphoid hypertrophy induced by the bacterial postnasal drip. It is not uncommon to see a septal deviation, particularly in the area adjacent to the middle turbinate. This deviation creates air turbulence that adversely affects sinus ostial function. Bacterial infection can also induce polyp formation; this can be purely bacterial or also may have an allergic component. Nasal cytology reveals polymorphoneucleocytes, bacteria, and intracellular bacteria. Rhinomanometry may or may not be normal. Typically, vasoconstriction does not alter nasal airflow. The CT scan will demonstrate the disease. Minimal disease will be seen solely in the ostiomeatal complex. More advanced disease may involve the maxillary sinuses, all of the ethmoid sinuses, and the frontal sinus. The sphenoid sinus is isolated and may or may not be involved. Without allergy, the IgE will be normal. Some individuals will have selective immunoglobulin deficiencies, and certainly if the history so dictates this should be looked for.

Initial treatment for a bacterial infection is prolonged use of antibiotics. Typically, the cilia have been so damaged that even though the sinus is sterilized with 1 or 2 weeks of antibiotic therapy, the cilia have not recovered and, therefore, the sinus is not functioning physiologically. Reinfection usually occurs in several days. Success depends not on the strength of the antibiotic but rather on its duration of use. Culture-directed antibiotic therapy is appropriate, but the key to success is the administration of an antibiotic for an extended period, such as 6 weeks of erythromycin 250 mg, four times daily, or doxycycline 100 mg, twice daily. One or two refills are indicated and the patients should be advised to take the antibiotics until they are well and then half again as long. Many patients do not get well for 5 to 8 weeks, and if it takes them 6 weeks to get well, they will need to continue the antibiotics for a full 9 weeks. If it takes them 8 weeks to get well they should continue to take it for the full 12 weeks.

ENDOSCOPIC SINUS SURGERY

If there is an allergic component to the disease, the judicious use of nasal steroids may facilitate opening of the ostiomeatal complex and for the most part, as long as the patient is protected with antibiotics, the use of nasal steroids is safe. If the antibiotic therapy fails, endoscopic sinus surgery is indicated, a relatively new but important development in paranasal sinus surgery. Using small endoscopes to look inside the nose, the surgery is directed at opening the natural drainage channels for the maxillary, ethmoid, and frontal sinuses. Older operations made new drainage channels that did not function physiologically and, did not perform with regular satisfaction. The new endoscopic sinus surgery is a more natural procedure, substantially less involved, and is performed under direct vision. It is not without risk, but it does add an element of safety. Abnormal and obstructive tissues are then removed using state-of-the-art microtele-scopes and instruments. In most cases, the surgery is performed entirely through the nostrils, leaving no external scars, little swelling, and only mild discomfort. Although in the past attention has often been directed toward the removal of all sinus mucosa from the major sinuses, the functional endoscopic approach relies on the principle that sinus disease is reversible if the underlying cause can be identified, corrected, and the natural sinus ostia enlarged to permit drainage of sinus secretions. A careful diagnostic work-up is therefore important and consists of endoscopic examination in the office, CT scans of the sinuses, nasal physiology (rhinomanomatry and nasal cytology), and selected blood tests.

This procedure takes practice to perfect, but it has become the procedure of choice when sinus surgery is required. It does the least harm, removes the least amount of tissues, and, unarguably, most effectively reestablishes the natural outflow of sinus secretions and the inflow of air.

Endoscopic sinus surgery can be performed under local or general anesthesia. The surgery is performed as an outpatient, meaning the patient goes home the same afternoon. The discomfort is minimal and far less than with the older, more conventional operations.

Potential surgical complications include bleeding, bruising around the eyes, swelling, scarring, and infection. Rare complications include the possibility of intracranial entry and spinal fluid leak. The ethmoid sinus is located under and adjacent to the brain, and the fluid that surrounds the brain can leak through the sinuses into the nose. There is then potential for infection that could result in meningitis. Because the endoscopes used in surgery allow improved visualization of the ethmoid sinuses, this complication is uncommon. Double vision and loss of vision have occasionally been reported after ethmoid surgery. Fortunately, they are rare complications.

The advantage of endoscopic sinus surgery is the philosophic recognition that the surgical goal is to open the natural drainage channels, thereby restoring normal physiologic function. This differs greatly from past procedures that were ablative and destructive. Other advantages over past sinus surgeries are diminished postoperative discomfort, minimal nasal packing, decreased bleeding, shortened recovery time, and most important, an improved success rate.

Because of potential bleeding problems, aspirin, Advil, and other NSAIDs must not be used for 10 days preceding and 10 days following surgery.

Light red to clear drainage from the nose is normal for 3 to 6 days following surgery. The outside gauze dressing needs to be changed when soiled or saturated. A 2 × 2 gauze pad folded in half over the nostrils and held in place with a strip of paper tape is sufficient.

Nasal packing is usually used after surgery. The nose should not be with packing in place. It is normal to have bad breath or smell a foul odor while the packing is in place.

Headaches and sinus or nasal discomfort are common after surgery. Pain relievers can be prescribed. Antibiotics and/or a moisturizing saline spray may be prescribed.

No swimming or strenuous activities should be attempted for at least 10 to 14 days after surgery, as this might produce bleeding or dislodge any packing that may be present. Diet should be normal. Alcoholic beverages should be avoided.

When directed, saline irrigations are recommended to reduce crusting and to keep sinus openings clear. We use 1 teaspoon salt in 1 quart warm water. Put this solution into a Water-Pik bowl (Water-Pik is a trade name for a dental cleaning device available at most drugstores for $35–$50). Using the Ethicore® Nasal Adaptor on the Water-Pik at settings between 1 and 2, the patient leans over a sink and irrigate both nasal passages. Irrigate twice a day, morning and evening.

ENVIRONMENTAL CONTROL
FOR ALLERGY

House Dust

House dust is partially composed of the breakdown products of natural plant and animal fibers. If these fibers or materials that make up a large part of the home furnishings (rugs, curtains, stuffed furniture, bedding, and so forth) are replaced with synthetic materials such as nylon, acetate, polyester, which are nonbiodegradable, much of the source of the house dust will be eliminated.

Bedroom

Because a large part of the time is spent in the bedroom, dust control in this area should be more vigorous. Remove stuffed or upholstered furniture. Any furniture should have smooth plastic, metal, or wood finishes. Remove from the room and the adjoining closet, all stored books, toys, clothing, bedding, and so forth that collect and produce dust. If some of these articles must be stored in the bedroom, they should be placed in plastic bags and sealed.

Bare wood or tile floors are best; if a rug seems necessary, washable throw rugs are recommended. Any rug should be 100% synthetic, and the pad should be foam or rubber. Curtains or drapes should be easily launderable and of synthetic material, although cotton is permissible.

Forced-air heater ducts leading to the bedroom should either be closed off or a polyester filter placed over the register. The central air filter should be replaced often during the winter months.

Bedding must be of synthetic material and laundered frequently. Avoid feather- or kapok-filled pillows. Mattresses and box springs should be covered by zippered, vinyl mattress covers, which may be purchased at most large department stores. The windows and doors leading to the bedroom should remain closed as much as possible. Initially, the walls, ceilings, and floors should be washed. Daily cleaning with a damp mop and a damp cloth is important.

Vacuums disperse large amounts of dust particles into the air; therefore, it is best to have the allergic person outside the home during and for at least 2 hours after running the vacuum cleaner. If the allergic individual does the vacuuming, a mask should be worn during this period.

Special Items

Pets, furry or feathered, should not be allowed in the home at any time. House plants should not be placed in the bedroom; the soil contains mold and biodegradable material that can be extremely allergenic.

Mold (mildew, fungi) is associated with damp places and can be eliminated or retarded by lowering the humidity via vents, fans, heaters, and so forth, and by using mold retardants such as Captan® (orthofungicide), which can be purchased at a local nursery. Zephiran® (benzalkonium cloride) 1:750, found in pharmacies, or some other commercially available mold retardants such as Lysol can also be used. Captan®, which is nonpoisonous to humans, may be sprayed through a garden spray; use 8 tablespoons of 25% solution or 4 tablespoons of 50% powder per gallon of water. Zephiran® (full strength) may be sprayed on walls and other areas.

Air cleaners or air purifiers are helpful. Portable units should be placed in the bedroom at a location where the clean air flow is across the head of the bed. Larger units are also available that can be incorporated with your existing forced-air heating system. There are two basic types of air cleaners on the market, a HEPA filter or an electronic air cleaner (electronic precipitator). Although both appear to work well, the HEPA filter is thought to be the more efficient of the two. Air cleaners may be rented to assess usefulness. Rental fees are usually applicable to sales price.

Because tobacco smoke is an irritant to the respiratory system, smoking should not be allowed in the home.

Many of the individuals presenting to the UCSD Nasal Dysfunction Clinic have a mixed inflammatory disorder. There is an allergic rhinitis and this is often the instigating problem. The disease is compounded by the growth of nasal polyps and then as one or another of the natural sinus ostia become obstructed, a bacterial infection ensues. Invariably the patient is also allergic to the bacterial infection and once the bacterial infection develops, the nasal disease worsens. These individuals are managed with both antibacterial and antiallergic treatments. It is common that they will require endoscopic sinus surgery to bring them back to some base level from which a purely allergic regimen can be instituted.

NASAL OBSTRUCTION

Nasal obstruction to those afflicted is a very annoying problem.

Case Study: Nasal Obstruction 1

A psychology student had such severe nasal obstruction that he was an obligate mouth breather. He had lived with this all his life but recently had met a new girlfriend who loved kissing. Because he could not breathe through his nose, he was having obvious problems. He denied any history of nasal injury and did not have any symptoms of nasal allergy. The external nose was straight with a rather prominent hooked dorsum. The septum was horribly crooked. I advised the patient that he would need a septoplasty to correct the breathing. I also told him that if he wished to have a rhinoplasty, this would be a good time, because the two operations should be done simultaneously. He eagerly requested both procedures. A septorhinoplasty was performed and a good functional and cosmetic result was obtained.

Various degrees of nasal obstruction occur and they rarely are all-or-none phenomena. Why does a patient with nasal obstruction suddenly decide to seek medical care? Sometimes the obstruction becomes noticeably worse or the patient becomes more aware of the problem. Once attention is focused on the obstruction, it can seem increasingly problematic. Patients who develop acute nasal obstruction from nasal trauma are also acutely aware of their problem and anxious to have it corrected. They may complain of a dry mouth or of an obstruction to breathing. History is the key to diagnosis. Which side of the nose is obstructed? Is it always obstructed or does the obstruction come and go? What brings it on, and what relieves it? An algorithm to approach nasal obstruction is shown in Figure 3.8.

The nose should be examined carefully. Unilateral obstruction is usually constant and implies an anatomic basis. This may be a foreign body, a nasal polyp, a nasal tumor, or most commonly, an obstructive nasal septal deviation. Bilateral obstruction can be caused by polyps, tumor, nasal septal deviation, or merely from drooping of the nasal tip associated with the aging process. Allergic rhinitis will also present as nasal obstruction. In this case, the obstruction is generally bilateral and will fluctuate. Many patients complain that when they lie down, one side of their nose becomes obstructed. It is always the lowermost or downside, and if they turn over, the nose clears and the other side becomes obstructed. This is a normal physiologic response, and the patient should be so advised. No treatment is necessary.

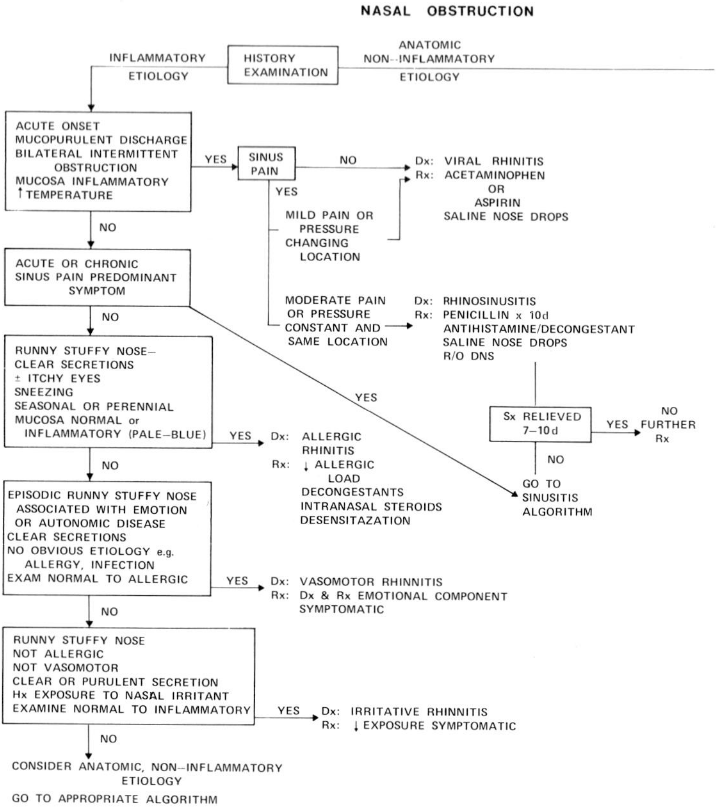

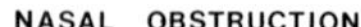

Figure 3.8.   Algorithm for the evaluation of nasal obstruction. *(Continued on p. 93.)*

The nose is a dynamic organ, responsible for filtering, warming, and humidifying inspired air and, to some degree, recapturing the humidity on expiration as well as preserving some of the heat. Because this is an intense process, the nose goes through a nasal cycle in which one side congests while the other side decongests. The decongested side is then responsible for the majority of the work, while the congested side has opportunity to rest. Most individuals cycle approximately four times a day. In some individuals, this normal nasal cycle is exaggerated or, at least, it comes to their attention and they find it to be bothersome. Those who complain to their physicians should be evaluated to rule out other problems such as anatomic obstruction or inflammatory disease. A good explanation will help patients understand what is happening, and will assure them that this is not a problem

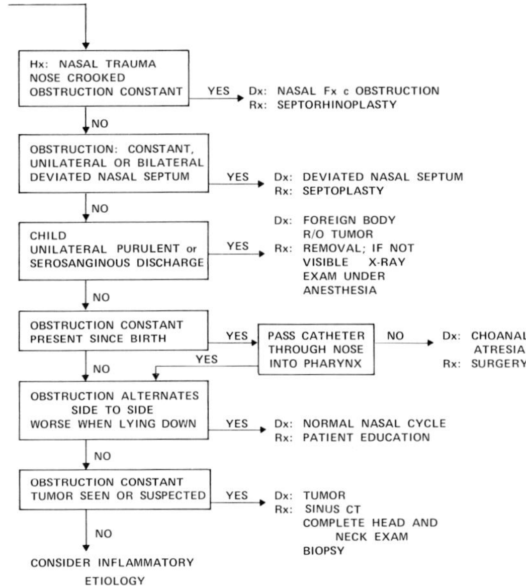

Figure 3.8.   (continued)

to be further pursued. The physician's responsibility is, of course, to recognize the normal nasal cycle and resist the temptation to treat with unnecessary surgery or medication.

Allergic rhinitis may also present with a runny nose. The common symptoms of allergic rhinitis are nasal obstruction, sneezing, tearing, and runny nose. The symptoms are seasonal or perennial. Allergic rhinitis may be associated with sinus disease and often occurs in conjunction with nasal polyps. The diagnosis is made initially by history. Examination reveals swollen, often bluish-purple mucosa covering the turbinates. A nasal smear will show eosinophils and/or basophils. Spraying the nose with 0.25% phenylephrine relieves the nasal obstruction. Nasal examination may reveal polyps, and sinus CT will indicate the extent of paranasal sinus involvement.

Case Study: Nasal Obstruction 2

A 7-year-old girl presented with a 5- to 6-month history of nasal stuffiness with a diminishing sense of smell and associated loss of appetite and resultant weight loss. She also complained of severe tiredness, and her mother noted some sluggishness. There were no other complaints, except a headache associated with a recent upper RTI. There was no family history of allergy, no history consistent with infection, and no history of nasal disease prior to the present illness.

Examination revealed a normal 7-year-old child. The anterior nares were filled with a mucoid material and it was impossible to see deeper into the nasal cavity. The oropharynx, oral cavity, and remainder of the head and neck examination were all within normal limits. A nasal work-up was initiated. Rhinomanometry revealed an infinite resistance in both nostrils; that is, the nose was totally occluded, even after it was sprayed with phenylephrine. Nasal cytology revealed a few polymorphonucleocytes and a few bacteria. The IgE was within normal limits, and the inhalant RAST panel was negative. A CT scan revealed a large cystic mass involving the mid-portion of the nasal cavity and nasopharynx. The mass was seen to bulge into the anterior cranial fossa, extending into the sphenoid sinus.

A neurosurgical consultation was obtained, which confirmed the history and physical examination. Her mental status, cranial nerves, motor, coordination, and gait examinations were all within normal limits. An MRI was obtained, which is shown in Figure 3.9. This revealed a large midline cystic lesion involving her sphenoid, with extension through the planasphenoidale into the frontal fossa. This latter extension was minimal; nonetheless, the gyrus rectus appeared to be elevated. The diagnostic impression was that this was a sphenoid sinus mucocele.

The patient was brought to the operating room where a sublabial approach to the nasal cavity was made. The cystic mass was easily identified. The fluid was evacuated, and the cyst dissected from the septum, nasopharynx, and superior nasal cavity. A small dehiscence in the clivus was noted, beneath and posterior to the pituitary. Dissection was completed using a microscope. The lesion was completely removed and there was no evidence of intracranial involvement. The frozen section diagnosis was a craniopharyngioma. This was confirmed on permanent evaluation.

The patient made an uneventful recovery with no neurologic, nasal, or endocrine dysfunction.

Occasionally, nasal secretion, stuffiness, or obstruction is more than just allergic rhinitis. In this case, it was a tumor that

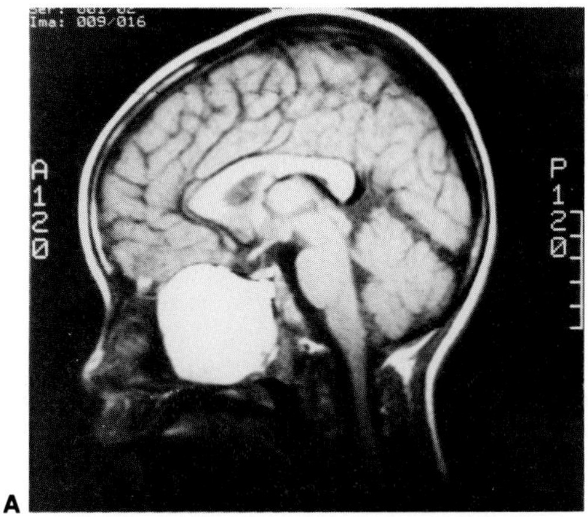

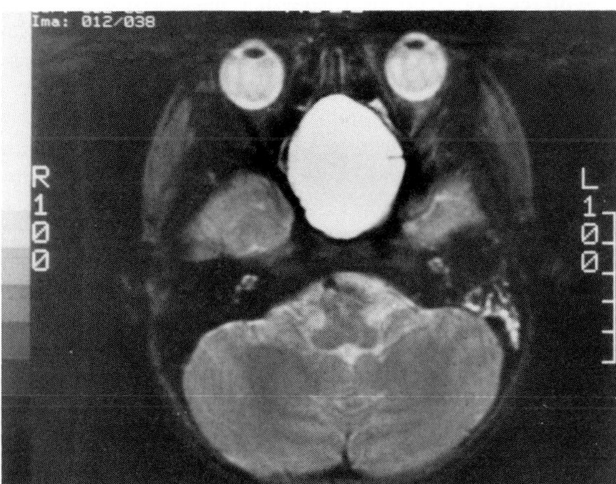

Figure 3.9. (A) T_1 magnetic resonance imaging (MRI) scan, sagital view, no contrast: high-signal intensity mass extending from clivus, sphenoid sinus, and floor of anterior cranial fossa. (B) T_2 MRI scan, axial view, no contrast: high-signal intensity mass occupying sphenoid sinus, posterior ethmoids, and posterior nasal airway.

was diagnosed before it eroded into and caused central nervous system disease. Once again, the necessity of a thorough work-up for patients with chronic, complex nasal dysfunction is shown.

RHINORRHEA

A runny or drippy nose is a common complaint. Frequently, it is a short-term problem often associated with an upper RTI. However, the runny nose can be a chronic condition. Table 3.3 lists the differential diagnosis for rhinitis. The diagnosis is generally made by a careful history and physical examination. Allergic evaluation and nasal cytology may help distinguish some causes. The algorithm shown in Figure 3.8 will help distinguish the causes of obstruction and discharge.

SMELL LOSS

The most important chemical sense is olfaction. It is currently estimated that 1% to 2% of the American population suffer from the loss of the sense of smell. For these $2\frac{1}{2}$ to 5 million individuals the world has lost some of its excitement. The most obvious and primary complaint is that food no longer has a taste, because, indeed, 95% of the sensory input received from food (and that that allows us to distinguish a good steak from a bad steak) is the sense of smell. But smell means a great deal more than just the ability to taste and enjoy food. First and foremost, it is a warning sign. Smoke is an early warning of fire. Most gasolines are odorized, and a gas leak is detected by its noxious mercaptan smell. Spoiled food smells horrible, and those without a sense of smell cannot protect themselves from poisoned food.

Table 3.3 Differential Diagnosis for Rhinitis

A. Acute viral upper respiratory tract infection (common cold)
B. Allergic rhinitis
C. Bacterial rhinosinusitis
D. Vasomotor rhinitis
E. Irritative rhinitis (tobacco, poor air quality, smoke, gases, chemicals)
F. Hormonal rhinitis (pregnancy, menstruation, endocrine)
G. Cold-induced rhinitis (skier's nose)
H. Gustatory rhinitis
I. Drug-induced rhinitis
J. Rule out CSF leak

RAST = Radio Allergo Sortent Test
CSF = CerebroSpinal Fluid

Smell is a major pleasure sense, and when one smells the fragrance of cut grass, of flowers, of the forest, of autumn, of spring, one derives not only information, but pleasure. We all know the smell of our loved ones. The sense of smell plays an important role in sexual excitement, and although Americans have done a great deal to camouflage body odor and sexual smells, they are still perceived and remain important. The sense of smell is necessary for body hygiene. How would one know when to change ones underwear or take a shower without the sense of smell?

The sense of smell, second only to hearing, is a strong component of memory. For example, the smell of cut grass brings back memories of childhood football, and the smell of grandfather's fishing vest brings back the smells of summer vacations. The smell of the kitchen brings back the smell of home, the smell of cooking brings the memories of festive holidays.

The loss of the sense of smell has not received the same attention that loss of vision and loss of hearing have, and hence, less is known about it, and patients know even less about what has happened to them. The nomenclature of smell is listed in Table 3.4 and includes definitions for anosmia, hyposmia, phantosmia, parosmia and presbyosmia.

The differential diagnosis for smell loss is long. The most important causes are described. *Inflammatory nasal disease* is responsible for approximately one third of the patients complaining of smell loss. Whether this is a chemical inhibition of olfactory epithelial function in the olfactory cleft or whether it represents a simple obstruction to air passage in the olfactory cleft is unknown. Inflammation can be caused by infection and/or allergy, if the inflammation is appropriately treated, the sense of smell can often be restored. *Head trauma* results in impaired sense of smell in approximately 10% of cases, particularly with frontal and occipital trauma. The brain is jarred relative to the cribriform plate, and the delicate olfactory nerves penetrating the crbriform are stretched or sheared. If stretched, the sense of smell returns, as in approximately one third of cases in which the majority recognize the returned smell within the first year posttrauma. If the nerves are sheared, olfaction does not return. These patients often experience phantosmias, much like a phantom limb complaint following an amputation. Another third of smell impairments are *post-*

Table 3.4 The Nomenclature of Osmia

Normosmia—A normal sense of smell
Anosmia—An absent sense of smell
Hyposmia—A diminished sense of smell
Parosmia—A distorted sense of smell
Phantosmia—A phantom sense of smell
Presbyosmia—Hyposmia associated with aging

viral in nature. Certain viruses, particularly of the influenza group, kill the olfactory epithelial cells and render the patient hyposmic. Once this occurs, there is no known treatment and prognosis for recovery is poor. Certain *toxins* are known to burn the olfactory epithelium. Ammonia is probably the most common, but other cleaning solvents have been reported as well. Some patients have a congenital loss of the sense of smell. For these individuals, the loss is not as great because it is a sense that they never had. The true incidence of congenital anosmia is not known, because many of the patients never complain and those that do are rarely reported. *Presbyosmia* is the loss of the sense of smell with aging. As the geriatric population increases, this becomes increasingly important, as there is no question that the sense of smell diminishes significantly with age. It diminishes faster in males and in those who smoke tobacco products. Certain *endocrine* dysfunctions are associated with smell impairment. The sense of smell is a primitive and basic sense and it is often associated with *psychiatric* illness. Some patients at a smell dysfunction clinic will, in fact, have a normal sense of smell and will have a mental health illness. There are many other causes, but the frequency of these is small.

The work-up begins with an olfactory test. Several are available. The most rudimentary is a scratch and sniff test. Sophisticated tests include olfactory-threshold and odor-identification testing. The work-up should also include an evaluation for abnormal physiology, which can include such tests as nasal cytology, rhinomanometry, and IgE and RAST screens. The examination must include a rigid endoscopic examination of the olfactory cleft and a sinus CT scan for paranasal sinus disease, olfactory cleft obstruction, and, occasionally, tumor.

For those with an inflammatory etiology, rigorous treatment can be prescribed. For all others, that is, those with a nonreversible cause, the patient is counseled. The most important counseling is that that educates the patient in the cause and reality that the sense of smell is, in fact, diminished or absent. Patient instructions are important for those with a diminished or absent sense of smell. They must have smoke detectors in all rooms in which they cook, burn fires, or sleep. Gas detectors must be present in all areas in which gases may be present, because if one is to light a match in a gas-filled room, the resultant explosion can be fatal. Because smell-impaired individuals cannot detect spoiled or rotten food, they must maintain a rather rigorous leftover-food discard schedule, and it is always best if their food is sniffed by someone with a normal sense of smell before they eat it.

Without question, the greatest loss is the pleasure derived from eating on social occasions. One invariably invites friends over for brunch, lunch, dinner, snacks, or "lets just eat anyway." In any case, food, its preparation, and its consumption are a major American pleasure. Rehabilitation in this regard is difficult. The patient may learn to focus on the other aspects of food, such as color, the presentation, and the texture, but these fall far short of the aromatic pleasures they once enjoyed. For some, the addition of hot trigeminal stimulants returns some interest in food. Pepper and curry are the two major hot trigeminal stimulants for food, and for many individuals, spicy Mexican or Indian food becomes interesting.

If little is known about olfaction, even less is known about taste. The chemical tastes on the tongue, modulated primarily by the seventh cranial nerve, are sweet, sour, salt, and bitter. The true incidence of chemical taste impairment is unknown. Although some purport it to be a large number with a complex work-up and a lengthy differential diagnosis, others consider this a rather infrequent problem and that those seriously concerned about their taste dysfunction generally have psychiatric rather than physiologic causes. Nonetheless, there are some physiologic problems that impair the sense of taste. Certainly, injury to the taste fibers in the ear at the chorda tympani or any site distal will alter the sense of taste. Certain drugs, such as metronidazole, will cause a metallic taste in the mouth, and although this is not truly a taste dysfunction, it is an abnormal taste, and fortunately one that disappears when the drug is discontinued. Many patients complain of an electric taste in their mouth. For some, this is caused by different metals used in dental restoration and thus a small battery is installed in the mouth. This is almost impossible to document and normally requires removing all the dental work and then redoing it with a single compound.

The sense of taste can be tested by applying sweet, salty, bitter, and sour compounds to the tongue. Intensity can also be measured but it is more difficult and requires a clinic setup to do so. For the majority who have lost their sense of taste, the impairment is small, and it may be that the majority never even come to medical attention because they adapt to the loss very quickly. Each patient deserves a work-up excluding tumors, gastric reflux, postnasal discharge, and obvious intraoral pathology. Psychiatric consultations should be obtained early, and the astute clinician should not pursue organic causes for a complaint that is most often psychogenic.

CHAPTER 4

The Throat: Oral Cavity, Oropharynx Larynx, Hypopharynx, Esophagus, and Trachea

A large number of diseases—both common and uncommon—affect the mouth, throat, larynx, and esophagus. It is difficult for a specialist to be conversant with all the diseases, and it would be extraordinary for a general practitioner to be familiar with all of them. Therefore, only the common maladies are discussed here. The practitioner should know the common diseases well and be able to treat them appropriately. Other diseases should be recognized as more complex and of a different nature; these should be referred to specialists.

TONSILLITIS

Tonsillitis is a common disease of children and young adults. It is an infection caused by bacteria, predominantly beta-hemolytic streptococci, involving the oropharyngeal tonsils, but also affecting the lymphoid tissues of the nasopharynx (adenoids) and the base of the tongue (lingual tonsils). Other organisms, including aerobes and anaerobes, can be cultured from tonsillar core tissue. The importance of their presence remains an important topic of discussion because if organisms other than streptococcus are the true pathogens, the antimicrobial therapy might be altered from penicillin to more potent antibiotics. Patients complain of an intense sore throat, which is often so sore that swallowing is painful. The tonsils can swell and cause dysphagia and may occasionally obstruct the airway. Patients will be febrile and look sick (toxic). Examination will verify an elevated temperature, usually above 101°F (39°C) in adults and greater than 103°F (40°C) in children. The tonsils are enlarged and often covered with white, exudative lymphoid tissue. The posterior pharynx, nasopharynx, nose, and larynx are all normal. Generally, there is significant anterior cervical lymphadenopathy. Many physicians will obtain bacterial cultures from the patient's throat. This is expensive and, unfortunately, is accurate only two thirds of the time. For both of these reasons, some physicians do not obtain a throat culture unless the patient has known cardiac valve disease or is immunologically suppressed. For these patients, there is a risk of sepsis or endocarditis, and a culture with sensitivity testing is potentially valuable. For all other patients in whom tonsillitis is suspected, treatment is given without obtaining cultures from the throat. Normally, 250 mg penicillin four times daily for 10 days is prescribed. Patients allergic to penicillin are treated with erythromycin. Most patients will be significantly better within 3 days. They must be encouraged to continue the treatment for the full 10 days. This is necessary to protect against glomerulonephritis and rheumatic heart disease.

Recurrent tonsillitis is often treated with a tonsillectomy. The current indications for tonsillectomy are elaborated in the section, "Tonsillectomy and Adenoidectomy: Indications and Problems," later in this chapter.

VIRAL PHARYNGITIS

Most people have one or two colds annually. The majority of these are viral infections affecting the mucosa of the upper respiratory tract. Symptoms begin with a sore throat and can be mild or intense, depending in part on the virus and in part on the host. The pain and inflammation can involve the larynx (laryngitis), the trachea (tracheitis), or the bronchi (bronchitis). Usually as the throat soreness disappears, the nose becomes congested. Initially, a clear rhinorrhea develops, but the discharge rapidly becomes purulent due to bacterial superinfection. Usually the paranasal sinuses are involved, and this is perceived as pain or pressure over the involved sinuses. Occasionally in adults, but frequently in children, the middle ear is also involved. At first the ear has a serous effusion, but this will often develop into a bacterial otitis media. Adults have low-grade fevers, and children tend to have higher temperatures. Breathing and swallowing are rarely compromised. Examination reveals diffusely inflamed pharyngeal and nasal mucosa. Purulence is rare. The inflammatory process includes the tonsils. Cervical adenopathy is usually present in children, less common in young adults, and most often absent in patients older than aged 30 years.

There is no specific therapy. Fluids, rest, vitamin C, and chicken soup have all been lauded as effective. Antibiotics are not effective against the viral inflammation but may be useful prophylactically against the sequelae of the bacterial superinfection. Older patients at risk for pneumonia are often treated with tetracyclines. Children who regularly develop otitis media should be treated with amoxicillin. Decongestants are useful to decrease the stuffy nose and sinus discomfort, and salt water gargle may alleviate the sore throat. Aspirin, or acetaminophen in children aged 12 years and less, decreases the temperature, malaise, and discomfort. Because histamine is not part of the nasal response to viral rhinitis, antihistamines are not indicated and may, in fact, adversely affect recovery.

PERITONSILLAR ABSCESS

A peritonsillar abscess, also known as PTA, is generally a mixed anaerobic infection of the space between the tonsil and the lateral pharyngeal wall. Its onset is rapid. Patients are febrile and show signs of toxicity. The pain, which is intense, is usually unilateral. Patients complain of dysphagia, may often drool, and may become dehydrated. Examination of the oral cavity is often difficult because of the trismus secondary to inflammation of the adjacent pterygoid muscles. The tonsil is unilaterally protuberant and the soft palate and uvula may be edematous.

Diagnosis is made clinically. The superior pole of the tonsil is anesthetized with 1% lidocaine and the abscess is then aspirated with an 18- or 20-gauge spinal or tonsillar needle. The abscess can be incised and drained under the same local anesthesia. The patient is hospitalized and IV therapy begun. Two million units of penicillin IV are given every 4 to 6 hours until results of specific sensitivity tests are available. The patient is discharged when he or she can swallow without difficulty. Culture- and sensitivity-directed oral antibiotics are continued to complete a full 10-day treatment.

Early PTAs may not require hospitalization. If the patient can swallow and if there are neither symptoms nor suspicion of a compromised airway, the abscess can be aspirated and the patient placed on oral antibiotics and observed at home. It is not unreasonable to aspirate a PTA twice, as long as the patient can swallow the antibiotics and maintain a reasonable fluid intake. Because otolaryngologists mostly see PTAs in an advanced stage, there is a tendency to be biased toward incision, drainage, and hospital admission. Primary care physicians and emergency department physicians tend to see these in an early stage so the treatment is more commonly aspiration as an outpatient. A good working relationship between the primary care provider and the specialist benefits all involved.

There is approximately a 10% risk of developing a recurrent abscess. Because the peritonsillar space has been obliterated by the previous infection, the abscess involves the adjacent parapharyngeal space. The carotid artery and jugular vein occupy the parapharyngeal space, and infection quickly involves these structures. Infection can spread inferiorly and involve the superior mediastinum. For these reasons, the patient is brought back to the hospital 6 weeks after the initial infection and an elective tonsillectomy is performed.

An alternate treatment is immediate tonsillectomy. This requires a positive diagnosis by aspiration. The patient is brought to the operating room, and the tonsils are removed under local or, preferably, general anesthesia. The patient is treated with IV penicillin, discharged when swallowing is possible, and continued on oral antibiotics for the complete 10-day therapy. The operation is more difficult in the acutely infected patient, but it seems to carry no significant risk and saves the patient an additional hospitalization, and thus may be preferable for advanced PTAs.

Not everyone agrees that the risk of a recurrent PTA is as high as 10%, nor that a tonsillectomy is indicated for all PTAs. Certainly, individuals with recurrent PTAs or those traveling to remote areas where advanced medical care may not be available should have a tonsillectomy. Otherwise, the physicians involved should make their recommendations and the patients should make their own informed decision.

Tonsillectomy and adenoidectomy (T&A) is a commonly performed operation. All physicians should be familiar with the indications, risks, and benefits of the procedures so they can better advise their patients who have tonsillar disease. A section fully describing current thinking about this operation appears at the end of this chapter.

DIFFERENTIAL DIAGNOSIS OF SORE THROAT

Many patients complain to their physicians of a sore throat. Not all sore throats are caused by streptococci or common viral agents. For this reason, one should be familiar with a more complete differential diagnosis. Figure 4.1 is an algorithm of the differential diagnosis for acute and chronic sore throat. The following is a differential diagnosis of a sore throat.

- Beta-hemolytic streptococcal tonsillitis may present as an intense disease with obvious physical findings, but it can also be less intense and have more subtle findings. It can be acute, chronic, or recurrent.
- Viral pharyngitis is clearly the most common cause of sore throat.
- Peritonsillar abscess is certainly less common than viral pharyngitis or streptococcal tonsillitis, but it is seen frequently. Unilaterality and severity are the keys to diagnosis.
- Mononucleosis can present with an intense pharyngitis. Both the tonsils and the pharynx are involved and will appear red and exudative. Usually, the history of increased need for sleep will indicate mononucleosis. The cervical lymphadenopathy, when present, is much greater than that seen with other infectious diseases. Diagnosis is by a positive mononucleosis spot test.
- Gonococcal pharyngitis presents as an intensely red pharynx; the patient has significant discomfort and dysphagia. Diagnosis requires obtaining a positive recent history of oral sexual contact and then a positive throat culture on chocolate agar. Gonococcus will not grow on the standard throat culture media.
- A variety of other infectious diseases may cause sore throat, including fungi, tuberculosis, diphtheria, and sexually transmitted disease. These are usually discovered when the sore throat shows unusual features or fails to improve with time with or without antibiotics. Specific cultures and an infectious disease consultation are useful. Immunologically compromised individ-

uals, including those with acquired immune deficiency syndrome (AIDS), often present with a sore throat or mouth. This is discussed in the chapter on AIDS. Tumors can also present as a sore throat and although they may be missed initially, must be seriously considered with persistent or recurrent sore throat.

Candida albicans can infect the oral cavity. A candidal infection is most often seen in children and diabetic patients, but it can occur in anyone taking antibiotics. There usually is a white exudate with a sensitive, hyperemic underlying mucosa. Microscopic examination and fungal culture of the scrapings are diagnostic. Oral candidiasis is treated with clotrimazole troches 10 mg po five times daily. The troche must be sucked and dissolved slowly because it is only truly effective while present in the mouth. This is normally prescribed for a 14-day period. If clotrimazole is not available, the oral candidiasis is treated with oral nystatin 500,000 U two or three times daily. A cherry-flavored oral nystatin preparation is available. Patients should swish it back and forth in their mouth for 5 minutes. Unfortunately, most patients swish for only 10 to 15 seconds and then swallow the medicine. Nystatin lozenges, as with the clotrimazole troches, are superior because they are sucked for several minutes. Patients should use the nystatin twice daily for 10 days. Patients prone to oral candidiasis can use oral clotrimazole or nystatin prophylactically. Fluconazole is a potent antifungal agent, albeit with potential side effects, that is effective in the treatment of severe head and neck candidiasis. It is used primarily in HIV-positive patients. The loading dose is 200 mg orally, followed by 100 mg orally, every day for 13 days.

- Recurrent herpes pharyngitis (aphthous stomatitis) is most common on the lip (cold sore), but it can occur elsewhere in the oral cavity. It may be associated with venereal herpes. Diagnosis is confirmed by the small, clear fluid-filled vesicles or the red-rimmed, tender, sessile, whitish ulcers left when the vesicles break. No specific therapy is available, but the discomfort can be treated. Liquid diphenhydramine hydrochloride is swished against the sore for several minutes. Milk of magnesia or a liquid antacid is then swished against the aphthous ulcer for several minutes. This treatment can be repeated hourly. If it does not affect cure after a week or so, the base of the ulcer can be injected with steroids. Normally the sores disappear within a week or so. Aphthous ulcers are more common in patients with suppressed immune systems, disseminated cancer, and patients on chemotherapy. Unfortunately, these patients recover much more slowly—the ulcers may linger for several weeks.
- Oral cavity and oral pharyngeal epidermoid cancers are found in patients with high tobacco exposure. The carcinogenic effect of tobacco is enhanced up to seven times by alcohol. Often these tumors are first noticed as a sore in the throat or mouth. They

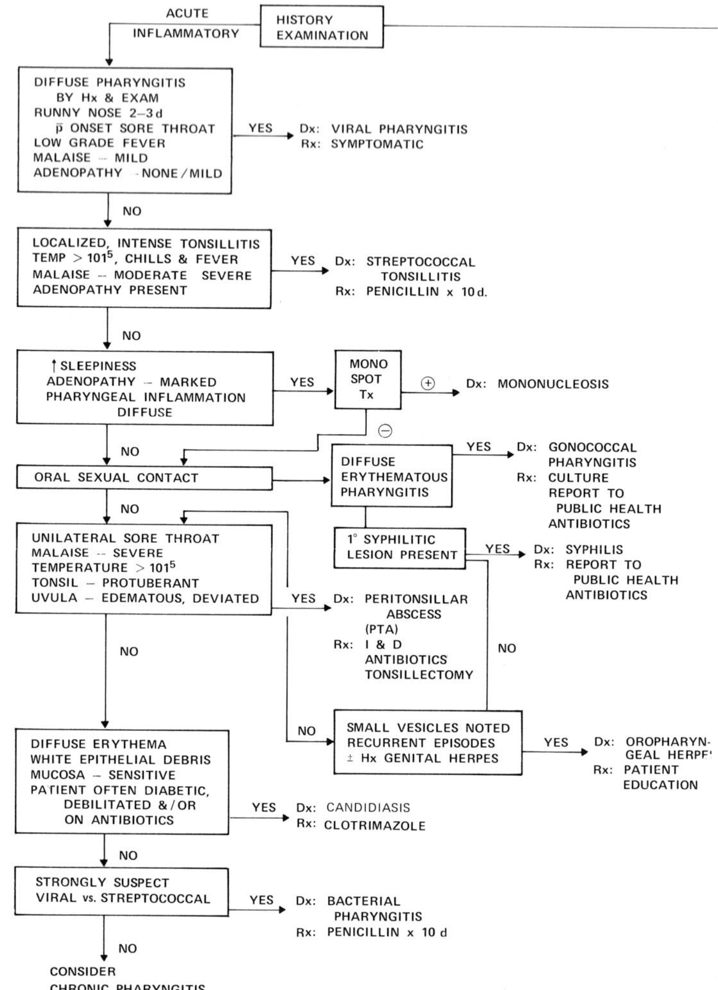

Figure 4.1. Algorithm for evaluation of acute and chronic sore throat. *(Continued on p. 107.)*

are painful, due to a bacterial superinfection. Many physicians fail to see the tumors and, instead treat their patients empirically with antibiotics. This temporarily alleviates the pain, but the pain recurs a week or two after stopping the antibiotics. Inevitably the pain is again treated with antibiotics and once again dissipates.

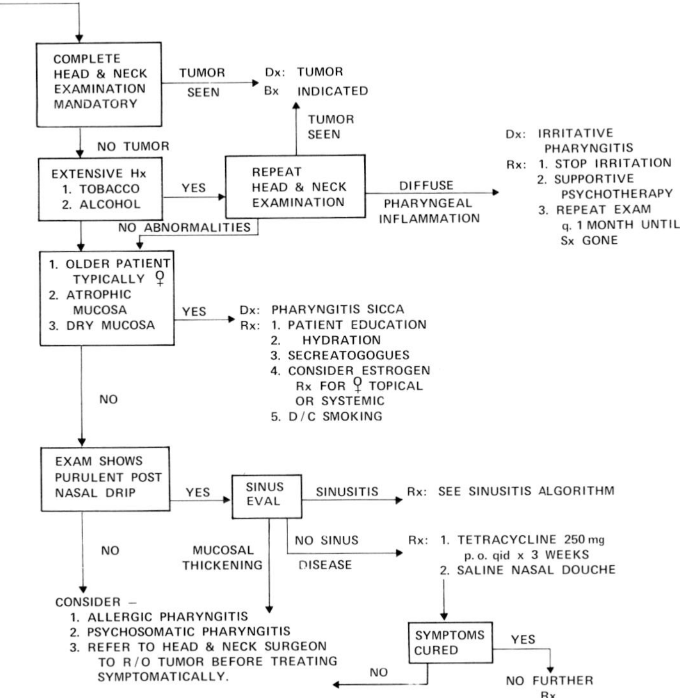

Figure 4.1. (continued)

This cycle can be repeated for months while the tumor grows. A tumor that was initially curable by local excision may become one that requires major extirpative surgery and one that has a much smaller chance of cure. Physicians must be suspicious of all mucosal sores, perform careful examinations, and look for these kinds of tumors. Oral neoplasms are discussed further in Chapter 6.

- Patients with allergic pharyngitis present with a mild, chronic sore throat. Examination may show some erythema and some lymphoid hypertrophy, but otherwise findings are unremarkable. A trial of antibiotics does not alter the symptoms. Saline gargle and other topical medicaments are also ineffective. Tentative diagnosis is made by exclusion of other etiologies. Generally, the allergy will be to isolated categories of foods. A careful history combined with experimentation by the patient will pinpoint the allergen. Treatment is exclusion of the offending allergen. Referral to an allergist is often useful.

- Both alcohol and tobacco damage the oral mucosa. When this causes symptoms of sore throat, it is called smoker's or drinker's pharyngitis, which present as a sore mouth, a sore throat, or both. Examination reveals a thinned, reddened, often dry mucosa. Treatment involves discontinuing or at least decreasing use of the offending substance. Unfortunately, patient compliance is poor, and the patient may return repeatedly with similar complaints. Neoplasm should be ruled out by careful examination at 1-year intervals.

- Pharyngitis sicca is a dryness of the mouth and throat caused by decreased salivary flow. Smoking, poor fluid intake, aging, mouth breathing, radiation therapy, and immunologic destruction of the salivary glands, as seen in Sjogren's syndrome, all predispose to a dryness of the mouth. A diagnosis can usually be made and specific treatment suggested. Nonspecific treatment includes increased hydration and the use of secretagogues, such as lemon drops.

ORAL CAVITY VENEREAL DISEASE

Because of the prevalence of oral sexual activity, an increasing number of patients are presenting with sexually transmitted diseases in the oral cavity. The most common infections are gonorrhea, syphilis, papilloma, and herpes. Other infectious diseases include chlamydial pharyngitis and trichomonal pharyngitis. Erythema, petechiae, and ecchymoses of the palate may be caused by fellatio. Tongue thrusting during cunnilingus often traumatizes the lingual frenulum. History is extremely helpful in diagnosing these maladies. An accurate history should be obtained openly and frankly. I usually say, "Sores like the one you have can be transmitted sexually. Have you had any recent oral sexual contacts?" Because the patient realizes the pertinence of the question, he or she will generally be honest.

Following are criteria for diagnosing the four most common sexually transmitted infections of the oral cavity.

- Gonorrhea presents as intense pharyngitis. Examination reveals a bright red throat. The differential diagnosis includes tonsillitis, mononucleosis, and viral pharyngitis. Diagnosis is suggested by recent oral sexual activity. Culture on specific media is diagnostic. Antibiotic treatment and referral to a public health service are mandatory.

- Syphilis presents primarily as a chancre on the mucosa of the oral cavity or oropharynx. The chancre is an ulcerative lesion and may or may not be painful. A positive oral sexual history can usually be obtained. Demonstration of the *Treponema pal-*

lidum and positive serology will confirm the diagnosis. Treatment includes antibiotics and referral to a public health service.

- Papillomas do occur in the nasal cavity and the oral cavity. Those associated with sexual disease (condyloma acuminatum) are found predominantly in the mouth and are usually multiple. A positive sexual history confirms the diagnosis. These lesions can be treated by cryotherapy or electrodesiccation. If either method fails, surgical excision is indicated. Podophyllin is not approved for the oral cavity and should not be used.
- Recurrent herpes pharyngitis, usually seen in females, is associated with genital herpes. It recurs in association with the genital herpes and is associated with both menstruation and stress. Diagnosis is best made by history, because the small, clear, fluid-filled vesicles are usually gone before the patient is seen by the doctor. No specific therapy is available.

SLEEP DISORDERS

Sleep disorders are now recognized as potentially dangerous and disabling problems. No single phrase refers to the group collectively but sleep apnea, obstructive sleep apnea, and sleep disorders are the most common. In the most severe cases, the patient experiences multiple apneic periods during sleep. Oxygen saturation falls and sleep is disturbed. A common complaint is daytime sleepiness because the patient never gets into deep sleep at night. With severe hypopnea, cardiac arrythmias can occur and occasionally induce cardiac arrest. Snoring is also considered a sleep disorder and may have a similar etiology as obstructive sleep apnea. Some individuals snore so loudly that no one can sleep with them; sometimes it is so loud no one can sleep in the same house.

Some cases of sleep apnea are controlled by the central nervous system. Others are caused by obstruction of air flow in the upper respiratory tract during inspiration. The evaluation of sleep disorders includes a good history, some of which may be supplied by a spouse. The patient can be monitored and an evening's sleep observed. Plethysmography records respiratory rate and apneic periods. Oxygen-saturation monitoring records the number of times the oxygen saturation falls below some arbitrary figure, such as 85%, and how long the patient spends with the oxygen saturation below that point. Another concern is how low the pO_2 falls. Oxygen saturations below 75% are considered moderately severe and those below 51% are considered severe. The electroencephalogram is also monitored and any arrythmia except premature ventricular contractions is of concern.

One of the causes of obstruction is obstructive nasal septal deviation. Also, large tonsils with a floppy, lax pharyngeal wall can collapse and literally obstruct the airway during inspiration. Similarly, a large tongue can fall posteriorly and obstruct the airway. In children, adenoids contribute to the airway obstruction.

Surgical correction includes septoplasty for septal deflections. Uvulopalatopharyngoplasty (UP3) resects the tonsils and adjoining lateral pharyngeal wall tissues, the uvula, and a portion of the soft palate. The pharyngeal and palatal wounds are closed, thereby tightening the pharynx, enlarging the nasal pharyngeal opening into the oropharynx, and decreasing oropharyngeal collapse and inspiratory obstruction during sleep. Overzealous surgery can result in unfortunate complications involving nasopharyngeal reflux of air, fluids, and even food. No uniformly successful procedures exist to correct posterior tongue obstruction.

In some severe cases, most commonly in the obese (pickwickian types), tracheostomy is required to bypass the upper airway during sleep. Tonsillectomy and adenoidectomy is commonly recommended in children with sleep disorders. The indications for these operations are not as precisely defined as they might be.

Other than monitors, continuous positive airway pressure and alarms, there is little medical management. Continuous positive airway pressure is an approach in which a mask is placed over the nose. During inspiration, positive pressure is provided by a bedside pump and the floppy obstructive airway is kept open. For some this is a cure—for others an objectionable, intolerable intrusion. As knowledge of these conditions increases, it is hoped that diagnosis and treatment will improve.

Snoring without other signs of sleep disorder is common. Those who sleep on their back need to learn to sleep on their side or stomach. If an occasional kick from a partner is not sufficient, a round sphere such as a tennis ball can be affixed to the rear of their sleeping attire between the shoulder blades. A tennis ball buttoned into a sewn-on pouch is perfect. When the patient rolls over on his or her back, the ball presses uncomfortably into the back and the patient immediately rolls back over.

If this fails to achieve satisfactory results, septal surgery and a UP3 can be considered. Often a sleep disorder clinic can help identify those who might benefit from surgical intervention.

GLOBUS HYSTERICUS

Globus hystericus is a common disorder. Patients complain of a feeling of fullness in the throat, a lump in the throat associated with swallowing, or a tightness in the throat. Sometimes, this is first noticed during an upper RTI and persists after all other symptoms resolve. The sensation is typically caused by a swollen epiglottis. As the swelling decreases, the patient remains aware of the epiglottis, which can be felt against the posterior pharyngeal wall with each swallow. The physician should explain this to the patient and suggest that ignoring the sensation will be helpful. Normally, the patient feels cured, and the physician then notices the presence of his or her own epiglottis for the next hour.

Persons under stress often develop a tightening in the throat. This spasm of the pharyngeal constrictors is clearly a psychosomatic disorder. In this case, it is the physician's responsibility to discover the stress and make the connection for the patient. The patient may then deal with the stress, either alone or with the aid of a professional (eg, physician, social worker, psychologist). Most physicians order a barium swallow, in spite of a classic history and a normal head and neck examination. This is rarely productive and is not indicated. If the history findings are not classic, a barium X-ray study is necessary to rule out other causes.

FOREIGN BODIES IN THE AIRWAY

Acute airway obstruction is not common, but it can be tragically fatal. It happens to young children, who frequently explore the environment by placing anything they can pick up into their mouths. Their oral and pharyngeal control is not fully developed. They lack the molar teeth to masticate potentially dangerous foods, such as peanuts. For all these reasons, young children are at serious risk for aspiration and airway obstruction. Older people with dentures who have had a little alcohol may lose oral sensation. They can chew a piece of meat and fail to realize it is poorly masticated. When they swallow, it fills the supraglottis and causes obstruction. This has been misnamed the *cafe coronary*. Complete obstruction presents as total airway obstruction and inability to talk or cry. The American Heart Association teaches the diagnosis and treatment of total airway obstruction in cardiopulmonary resuscitation (CPR) courses. The universal signal for obstruction is a hand placed in front of the neck. The rescuer asks the victim, "Can you breathe?" "Can you talk?" If the victim shakes his head "No," the Heimlich maneuver, or artificial cough, is given. Although techniques differ slightly, the basic theory and maneuver are the same. The rescuer's hands are gripped together over the epigastrium. The thoracic cage is stabilized with the rescuer's arms. The abdomen is rapidly compressed. With the chest held rigid, a rapid increase in abdominal pressure forces the diaphragm superiorly and rapidly increases the intrathoracic pressure. The foreign body that is lodged in the airway is literally popped out, just as a cork is popped out of a cork gun. This technique has now been used successfully in thousands of cases and should be known not only to physicians but to all safety-conscious people. Its use and complications are fully elucidated in American Heart Association literature.

Partial obstruction involves inspiratory and expiratory stridor, a high-pitched respiratory sound associated with a partial obstruction of the airway. Patients with this problem are kept in a comfortable position (usually sitting up) and transported as rapidly as possible to the emergency department and then to the operating room, with an anesthesiologist and a head and neck surgeon in attendance. The patient is anesthetized and the foreign body removed. Children will often aspirate the foreign body into the trachea or bronchi. This initially causes severe coughing. The cough then stops rapidly and the patient looks and feels well, which can engender a false sense of security. The patient should have a chest X ray. Nonopaque foreign bodies can sometimes be seen by taking inspiratory and expiratory right and left lateral decubitus chest X rays. Air trapping suggests an obstruction. All patients with foreign bodies in the airway must undergo a diagnostic bronchoscopy and removal of the foreign body. If a foreign body is present but not removed, a tremendous inflammatory process begins and within several days pneumonia will develop. At such time bronchoscopic removal of the foreign body is difficult or impossible; thoracotomy may be required.

When there is any clinical suspicion of a foreign body, immediate bronchoscopy is strongly advised. Waiting can be disastrous.

FOREIGN BODIES IN THE ESOPHAGUS

Esophageal foreign bodies are found in all age groups. They occur for two reasons. First, if a sharp, still object such as a needle, fish bone, or chicken bone is swallowed, it can stick anywhere from the oropharynx to the lower esophageal sphincter. If a foreign body is swallowed and reaches the stomach, it is rare for it not to pass on through the rest of the gastrointestinal tract and be expelled. However, any foreign body sticking in the esophagus must be removed, because it will not advance farther but, rather, will erode through the mucosa and cause a serious local infection, such as mediastinitis.

A second cause of a foreign body is an inherent esophageal obstruction. This can be a tumor, cricopharyngeal muscle spasm, esophageal diverticulum, posterior mediastinal mass (either a tumor or a vascular anomaly), enlarged left atrium as in congestive heart failure, or some abnormality of the lower esophageal sphincter. These obstructions can block the passage of a normal-size food bolus but mostly involve a large bolus, such as a piece of meat. Symptoms vary, depending on location. Pain is often felt and is usually described as a sensation of something being stuck. The patient is unable to eat any additional food. Diagnosis is by history and is confirmed by soft tissue X ray and a barium swallow, often with cinefluroscopy. Once the diagnosis is certain, the patient is anesthetized and the foreign body is located by esophagoscopy and removed, generally by a head and neck surgeon.

Fiberoptic bronchoscopy and esophagoscopy recently have become commonplace diagnostic tools. They are extremely effective when used for appropriate diagnostic procedures, but are potentially harmful in the diagnosis and treatment of disorders caused by foreign bodies, because they can injure local tissue and frequently are ineffective for foreign body extraction. For these purposes, rigid endoscopy is safer and provides the surgeon with a much greater chance to remove the foreign body. Using a fiberoptic instrument for diagnostic purposes can make removal more difficult.

Another common tragedy is that of young children drinking caustic materials, either acids or, more commonly, basic cleaning solutions, such as lye or drain cleaner. Diagnosis is confirmed by endoscopy, which must be done by a skilled surgeon with a rigid esophagoscope. Treatment consists of hospitalization, IV penicillin, and systemic steroids. Esophageal rupture and stricture are significant risks. For all of these maladies, an ounce of prevention is worth a pound of cure. Parents must be continually advised to keep easily swallowed objects and caustic materials locked away or otherwise out of reach of children.

Case Study: Foreign Body in the Esophagus

The following case was attended by and is presented with the permission of Dr. Wilfred Morioka, Clinical Associate Professor of Surgery, University of California Medical Center, San Diego. It is somewhat extraordinary but highlights some important principles of managing a foreign body. The patient was a young navy recruit who was at sea. When the ship passed from the harbor to the open seas, a heavy storm struck and the boat began rolling. The recruit became seasick. He was, unfortunately, unable to vomit. A sympathetic friend recommended induction of vomiting by sticking a finger down the throat. The recruit decided that rather than getting his hand dirty he would use something else. He made a loop in a coat hanger and shoved this down his threat. He vomited immediately, but unfortunately the force of the wretching impaled the bared end of the wire into his esophagus. He reported to the infirmary with a piece of wire sticking out of his mouth. Posteroanterior and lateral X rays from this patient are shown in Figure 4.2. The wire was removed endoscopically.

HOARSENESS

Changes in voice are common complaints and often frightening to patients, for they are a well-known sign of cancer. The usual change is a roughness to the voice. Less common is a breathy sound to the voice. Diagnosis is made by examination of the larynx with a mirror placed at the back of the throat. Although any practicing physician should be able to do this, head and neck surgeons have the most expertise. The four most common problems are laryngitis, vocal cord nodules, vocal cord paralysis, and laryngeal cancer.

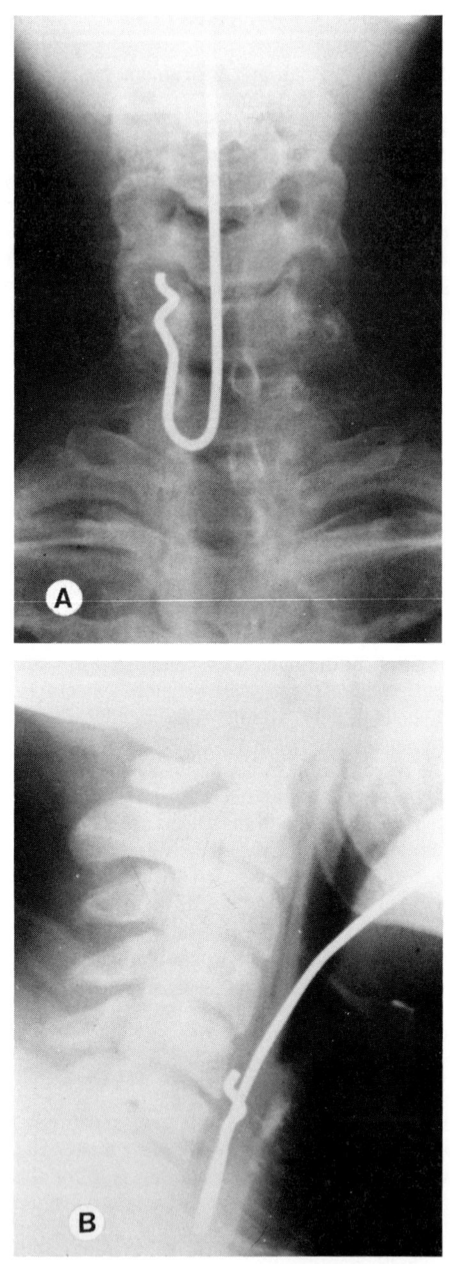

Figure 4.2. X rays of a coat hanger impaled in the cervical esophagus. (**A**) Posteroanterior view. (**B**) Lateral view.

Acute viral laryngitis is an inflammatory swelling of the vocal cords associated with an acute upper RTI. The same process seen in the posterior pharyngeal mucosa involves the vocal cord mucosa. Antibiotics are not effective. Patients should be cautioned to use their voices softly and sparingly. Abuse may cause scarring and a permanent hoarseness. Another classic history involves the sports fan who presents on Monday morning with no voice at all. History reveals such patients "yelled their heads off" at some sports event. Examination reveals inflamed vocal cords, called acute traumatic laryngitis. Again, the only treatment is voice rest. Both of these conditions improve over 7 to 14 days. If they do not, consultation with a head and neck surgeon is indicated.

Vocal cord nodules are small scars on the vocal cords. They usually occur in pairs and produce a rough, raspy voice. In children and mothers, they are called screamer's nodules, because this is exactly how they originated. Acute laryngitis can cause similar scarring, especially in patients who have not rested their voices during the recovery period. Endotracheal intubation can also cause this kind of vocal cord damage. Diagnosis is made by mirror laryngoscopy. Early nodules may resolve with voice rest. Speech therapy may also help. If the nodules do not regress with rest and voice therapy, a direct laryngoscopy is indicated. Under microscopic control the nodule is carefully dissected from the vocal cord. The patient must then observe absolute voice rest for 2 weeks. Follow-up voice therapy is mandatory for patients who abuse their voices.

Vocal cord paralysis presents with a breathy voice. The paralysis may be due to trauma, laryngeal cancer, or thyroid cancer. The left recurrent laryngeal nerve loops around the aortic arch and, because of this superior mediastinal disease or cardiac dilatation, can cause left vocal cord paralysis. Vocal cord paralysis is occasionally seen as a congenital lesion. Diagnosis is confirmed by mirror laryngoscopy, but in all cases a complete work-up includes laryngoscopy and biopsy of any suspicious lesion, examination of the neck, thyroid scan, and chest X ray. For left vocal cord paralysis without evidence of laryngeal or cervical disease, CT examination or MRI of the superior mediastinum is indicated. Assuming the appropriate cause has been discovered and treated, a variety of operations can be performed to improve the patient's voice. Tracheostomy is rarely indicated for a unilateral vocal cord paralysis, but it is mandatory for a bilateral vocal cord paralysis.

Case Study: Hoarseness

This case example highlights the evaluation made by a speech therapist for a 40-year-old male who presented with hoarseness following a heavy teaching load. He had a history of recurrent sore throats and had had a husky voice for the preceding 2 years, all of which had been related to his teaching schedule. He was currently carrying a heavy teaching load about which he was quite concerned. He was not taking any medication. The only pertinent findings of the physical examination were two small symmetrical vocal cord nodules, which were clearly causing this man's vocal changes.

The speech therapist's initial evaluation was summarized as follows: The patient denied respiratory problems and shortness of breath. He did have episodes of fatigue after talking to his class for an entire period. He could sustain a phoneme /a/ for 27.2 seconds and /ee/ for 33.5 seconds. Both of these were above the normal duration for this man's age and sex. The difference in sustained vowels suggested a constriction of the larynx with reduced air flow for both sounds. The patient demonstrated upper thoracic breathing and tended to release air prior to phonation or, occasionally, to hold back air during phonation. The patient spoke at approximately G-sharp^2, which is at the lower end of average for an adult male. His phonational range was approximately two octaves, from D-sharp^2 to F^4. However, he did not use adequate vocal variation during his conversational speech. A hard glottal onset was noted for most vowels. This was often preceded by a burst of air, indicating poor glottal approximation following inhalation. The patient's voice did not resonate normally and appeared to be primarily tense, with a strained, strangled quality. There were episodes of breaks into breathiness. His projection was constricted at the laryngeal level. He had difficulty increasing loudness.

The speech therapist's impression was of a long-term voice misuse with vocal hyperfunction. Therapy consisted of excessive voice reduction and initiation of a voice therapy program designed to improve the patient's respiratory/phonatory coordination. The patient underwent several weeks of intense therapy consisting of two 1-hour sessions a week, with a dramatic improvement in his voice. Over a period of 3 months, the vocal cord nodules disappeared and the patient's voice returned to normal.

Unfortunately, the patient presented again a year later after noticing some voice changes. Consultation was sought with the speech therapist and in two sessions, the patient's voice was tuned back to its normal state. From that point, the patient had a consultation with the speech therapist every 6 months, maintained his teaching load, and remained well.

Laryngeal cancers are usually epidermoid neoplasms associated with tobacco use. The voice has a rough, raspy sound, and the diagnosis is strongly suspected by the positive history of tobacco use and the insidious onset of hoarseness. Mirror laryngoscopy confirms the diagnosis. A full work-up should include complete blood cell count, urinalysis, determination of creatinine, bilirubin, and alkaline phosphatase levels, chest X ray, and neck examination. A direct laryngoscopy is performed and the tumor is biopsied. These tumors are best evaluated and treated by head and neck surgeons. The specific modes of therapy will be discussed in a later section.

Another common cause of hoarseness, cough, and a repeated need to clear ones throat is postnasal drip. The postnasal drip is usually caused by an indolent chronic rhinosinusitis, but can be induced by allergic rhinosinusitis as well. The secretions that drain down the posterior and lateral pharyngeal walls irritate the arytenoids and posterior larynx. This induces the cough and constant clearing of the throat. With prolonged irritation, the vocal cords become irritated and edematous and the voice develops a hoarse quality.

Examination will generally confirm posterior or lateral oropharyngeal irritation. Laryngeal examination will reveal the edema and erythema of the posterior larynx and vocal cords. Treatment is directed at evaluating, diagnosing, and treating the rhinopathy.

ACUTE EPIGLOTTITIS

Acute epiglottitis, also known as supraglottitis, is an infection of the supraglottis caused by *H. influenzae*. Patients are usually between 3 and 5 years old, but the disease does affect younger children and adults as well. Patients are generally febrile and show toxic symptoms; sometimes they drool because of the pain when they swallow. The frequency of signs and symptoms is given in Table 4.1. The supraglottis becomes edematous and the airway narrows. The patient rapidly

**Table 4.1 Frequency of Symptoms
and Signs of Acute Epiglottitis**

	(%)
Symptoms	
Fever	100
Respiratory distress	100
Sore throat	60
Dysphagia	60
Stridor	50
Irritability or restlessness	50
Drooling	40
Cough	35
Hoarseness	25
Signs	
Cyanosis	25
Retractions	20

develops inspiratory stridor. As the swelling progresses, the patient rapidly has increasing difficulty in swallowing. Examination commonly reveals a toxic febrile child, usually with some degree of inspiratory stridor. Pharyngeal examination may show a red, swollen epiglottis, but care should be taken when looking for this. Touching the epiglottis with the tongue blade may induce fatal laryngospasm. The patient is often most comfortable sitting up. The diagnosis is made by the clinical picture. Soft tissue lateral X rays may show the swollen epiglottis and confirm the diagnosis. However, as airway obstruction may occur at any time in patients with epiglottitis, a child with any suspicion of epiglottitis should never be sent to X ray unless attended by a physician skilled in intubation. If blood cultures are taken, they often grow *H. influenzae*.

Treatment must be immediate. Humidified mask oxygen should be started. Racemic epinephrine inhalation may greatly improve breathing. Dexamethasone or methylprednisolone and ampicillin should be given intravenously. Mild cases can be observed in an intensive care unit where a physician is readily available to intubate the patient. A patient who begins to improve can generally go to the ward the following day and be discharged the next. Patients with more severe cases should be brought directly to the operating room with an anesthesiologist, pediatrician, and a head and neck surgeon in attendance. If the anesthesiologist can intubate the patient, this is sufficient; if not, an emergency tracheostomy will be necessary. The patient is then watched in an intensive care unit and the tube is removed at 72 hours. A 7- to 10-day course of antibiotics (ampicillin IV and then amoxicillin orally) is necessary for all patients. Systemic steroids are discontinued as soon as the patient's airway is secure.

There are two additional diseases that must always be included in the differential diagnosis of acute epiglottitis. Croup is the most common cause of acute infectious respiratory problems in children. Generally a viral tracheitis, with or without involvement of the larynx, it typically occurs in children between the ages of 1 and 3 years and is preceded by a viral upper RTI. The child with croup wakens during the night with acute respiratory difficulty and classic inspiratory stidor. Most cases can be treated at home; the child is picked up, and allowed to breathe warm, humidified air, typically obtained by turning the shower on as hot as possible and holding the child at the entrance to the shower so that he or she can breathe the hot, humid air. The child can then be put back to sleep. The room air should be humidified with a humidifier, readily available at drugstores and similar shops. Occasionally, croup can be extremely severe; these cases require hospitalization and sometimes even intubation to maintain an airway. At times, a bacterial infection can invade the trachea, and the patient will require hospitalization and antibiotics.

Subglottic stenosis can occur as an idiopathic growth problem, as the sequela of endotracheal intubation, or as a result of subglottic hemangioma. It will often present as an acute inspiratory airway problem and may be associated with an acute upper RTI. It must be differentiated from croup and epiglottitis. The children present primarily with a moderate to severe respiratory difficulty but with no other signs of infection. Soft tissue posteroanterior and lateral X rays of the larynx and trachea will show the subglottic stenosis. Often bronchoscopy is required to confirm the diagnosis. The prognosis and treatment for subglottic stenosis depends on its etiology and its severity.

TONSILLECTOMY AND ADENOIDECTOMY: INDICATIONS AND PROBLEMS*

Approximately 750,000 Americans undergo tonsillectomy and adenoidectomy T&A each year, incurring a cost approaching $ one billion annually. The first combined T&A procedure was recorded in 3000 B.C. and yet with 5 thousand years' experience, there is still strong controversy regarding the risks and benefits of one of the most common surgical procedures. The indications for adenoidectomy, tonsillectomy, or combined T&A vary from life-threatening illnesses to problems of only minor disability.[1] Similarly, the risks vary from minor to major. In an effort to place these variables in proper perspective, the current indications for and complications in carrying out a tonsillectomy, adenoidectomy, or combined T&A will be discussed.

Surgical Indications

It must first be understood that there are no absolute circumstances for any surgical procedure, but there are very strong indications. For a tonsillectomy they are as follows:

- Carcinoma of the tonsil can occur in any age group. Lymphoma can be found in the tonsil in young and older adults, and epidermoid carcinoma of the tonsil is seen in patients with long smoking and drinking histories. Biopsy is necessary for diagnosis and the best technique for biopsy, staging, and control of bleeding requires complete removal of that tonsil. Contralateral tonsillectomy is not necessary.
- Peritonsillar abscess is caused by a bacterial infection, most often anaerobic in nature. If fine-needle aspiration (FNA) is not sufficient, incision and drainage is mandatory to prevent extension of the infection into the space around the carotid artery. Incision and drainage, along with appropriate antibiotic therapy, is curative for an acute episode. Approximately 10% of peritonsillar abscesses recur, and because of the destruction of the peritonsillar

*This section from Davidson TM, Calloway CA: Tonsillectomy and adenoidectomy. West J Med 133:451–454, 1980. Reprinted with permission.

space by the first abscess, a recurring abscess may extend rapidly into the parapharyngeal space and may quickly be fatal. Therefore, it is considered wise to carry out a tonsillectomy for peritonsillar abscess. This may be done either at the time of the initial discovery of the abscess or by elective surgery 6 weeks later. This is a decision that should be made jointly by the patient and surgeon.

- Congestive heart failure is sometimes seen in young children. This can be caused by a persistent upper airway obstruction and it presents as a heart failure of the right side. The airway obstruction is most commonly caused by the tonsils. Tonsillectomy, usually in association with adenoidectomy, will alleviate the airway obstruction and reverse the entire cardiac process.[2]
- Sleep disturbances in children and adults are frequently recognized. This can present as restlessness during sleep, snoring, or sleep apnea. In children this can be caused by large obstructive tonsils. Tonsillectomy and adenoidectomy is often recommended as the first step in the treatment of pediatric sleep disturbance. For adults, tonsillectomy or a UP3 may be recommended.
- Acute tonsillitis is sometimes so severe that respiratory difficulties and significant dysphagia develop, requiring hospitalization. Any episode of tonsillitis causing respiratory embarrassment or dysphagia so severe that hospitalization is required is best treated by elective tonsillectomy 6 weeks after resolution of the tonsillar infection.

The two most common philosophic indications for tonsillectomy involve decisions that must be made by both patient and physician. The first, recurrent tonsillitis, is a very elusive disease.[3] Many patients have a history of multiple episodes of recurrent tonsillitis, usually 6 to 12 or more per year. However, this is difficult to document. Often if these patients are followed closely, they may have far fewer episodes per year. In addition, evidence of a bacterial tonsillitis as opposed to a viral RTI is difficult to document. The entire picture is confused by the inaccuracies of the common throat culture streptococci and other bacteria. Nonetheless, it is currently believed by most otolaryngologists that a patient having four or more episodes of bacterial tonsillitis a year for at least 2 years that necessitates missing 10 or more days a year of school or work will benefit by tonsillectomy. This is a philosophic decision—one that the patient or guardian must ultimately make after he or she understands the risks and potential benefits of that procedure.

Many physicians believe that recurrent otitis media is another important indication for tonsillectomy. Although this is not always so, in some patients, an upper RTI occurs and progresses into serous otitis media and ultimately acute suppurative otitis media. If these infectious conditions cannot be successfully treated with antibiotics, then T&A may be warranted to prevent recurrent acute otitis media.

The physician might be particularly swayed in this direction if acute otitis media always resolves into a long bout of serous otitis media associated with a conductive hearing loss.

Adenoidectomy is strongly indicated in young patients with severe obstruction of nasal airways. This is often associated with hyponasal speech and tongue thrust with maxillary dental protrusion.[4] Although

Table 4.2 Current Indications for Tonsillectomies and Adenoidectomies

Tonsillectomy—strong indications
1. *Carcinoma of the tonsil.* The best technique for optimal results from biopsy and staging requires complete removal of the tonsil.
2. *Peritonsillar abscess (PTA).* A bacterial abscess, PTA is most often caused by anaerobic organisms. Incision and drainage is mandatory. Recurrent abscess rate is 10% and recurrent abscess may be fatal. Therefore, the tonsil should be removed. This may be done at the time of the initial PTA presentation or may be done electively 6 weeks later.
3. *Congestive heart failure.* Failure of the right-side of the heart can be caused in young children by a constant upper airway obstruction. This is reversed by tonsillectomy.
4. *Tonsillitis causing respiratory difficulties, dysphagia, and requiring hospitalization.* Any episode of tonsillitis causing respiratory embarrassment, or so severe that hospitalization is required, is best treated by elective tonsillectomy 6 weeks after the episode.

Tonsillectomy—philosophic indications
1. *Recurrent tonsillitis.* It is currently believed by most otolaryngologists that a patient having four or more episodes of tonsillitis a year for at least 2 years that necessitates their missing 10 or more days a year of school or work will benefit from a tonsillectomy.
2. *Sleep disturbances.* Sleep apnea, sleep disturbance, and snoring can be caused by upper respiratory tract lymphoid tissues that prolapse into and obstruct the airway during sleep. In these cases, tonsillectomy, adenoidectomy, and even partial palatectomy with uvulectomy (UP3) may improve the airway.
3. *Recurrent otitis media.* In some patients acute otitis media always or frequently develops following upper respiratory tract infections. If these cannot be successfully treated prophylactically with antibiotics, beginning at the onset of the upper respiratory tract infection, it may be an indication for T&A.

Adenoidectomy—strong indications
1. *Nasal airway obstruction.* This is often associated with hyponasal speech and tongue thrust with maxillary dental protrusion. Few patients should have adenoidectomy for the latter reasons alone, but the few that should will benefit.

(continued)

Table 4.2 Continued

Adenoidectomy—philosophic indications
1. *Recurrent tonsillitis.* A prepubertal patient with recurrent
   streptococcal tonsillitis who is to be treated by tonsillectomy should
   have adenoidectomy at the same time.
2. *Chronic otitis media with effusion.* Some cases of chronic otitis
   media with effusion also called serous otitis media, recurrent or
   persistent, may be cured by adenoidectomy. To date, no one knows
   how to select those who will benefit from this operation. Therefore,
   patients with prolonged serous otitis media associated with a
   conductive hearing loss or retraction of the tympanic membrane or
   both should have myringotomy with insertion of middle ear
   ventilation tubes. If they have large adenoids, documented by a soft
   tissue lateral X ray study or nasal obstruction, adenoidectomy may
   be of significant benefit. If the patient has large tonsils and
   recurrent tonsillitis particularly predisposing to ear infections,
   tonsillectomy should be carried out as well.

Table 4.3 Tonsil and Adenoid Surgery*

I. Indicators (one of the following)
  A. Obstruction of airway not associated with other conditions
    1. Tonsillectomy and/or adenoidectomy
      a. Suspected tonsil or adenoid hypertrophy with
        obstruction
      b. Sleep apnea and/or severe sleep disturbances
      c. Cor pulmonale—not solely attributed to other causes
      d. Failure to thrive—not solely attributed to other causes
      e. Obligate mouth breathing—not solely attributed to
        other causes
      f. Eating or swallowing disorders—not solely attributed
        to other causes
      g. Speech abnormalities—not solely attributed to other
        causes
    2. Chronic otitis media with effusion (secretory otitis media)
      persisting after adquate medical therapy
    3. Recurrent otitis media persisting after adequate medical
      therapy
    4. Chronic or recurrent purulent nasopharyngitis persistent
      after adequate medical and/or immunotherapy
    5. Recurrent or chronic otitis media with perforation and
      recurrent otorrhea complicated by suspected
      nasopharyngeal obstruction and/or nasopharyngitis
      persisting after adequate medical therapy
    6. Suspected adenoid hypertrophy
  B. Obstruction of upper airway associated with other causes
    1. Tonsillectomy and/or adenoidectomy
      a. Suspected orofacial anatomic abnormalities resulting in
        narrowed upper airway

Table 4.3 Continued

---

    b. Dental growth abnormalities
    c. Cardiac disease exacerbated by the upper airway obstruction
    d. Chronic otitis media

C. Infection
  1. Tonsillectomy
    a. Recurrent tonsillitis despite adequate medical therapy
    b. Recurrent tonsillitis when complicated by:
      (1) Peritonsillar abscess
      (2) Peritonsillar abscess with extension into adjacent tissue spaces
      (3) Abscessed cervical nodes
      (4) Acute airway obstruction
      (5) Febrile seizures
    c. Recurrent tonsillitis when associated with other conditions
      (1) Cardiac valvular disease with recurrent streptococcal tonsillitis
      (2) Recurrent otitis media
    d. Recurrent tonsillitis when associated with a persistent pathogenic streptococcal carrier state
      (1) Nonresponsive to adequate medical therapy
      (2) A noncompliant patient or noncompliant responsible adult
    e. Recurrent tonsillitis when associated with persistent chronic tonsillar inflammation and
      (1) Chronic intermittent sore throat not solely attributable to other causes
      (1) Halitosis related to tonsillar cryptic debris
  2. Adenoidectomy
    a. Chronic or recurrent purulent nasopharyngitis despite adequate medical and/or immunotherapy
    b. Recurrent acute otitis media or otitis media with effusion complicated by nasopharyngeal obstruction and/or nasopharngitis despite adequate medical therapy
    c. Recurrent or chronic otitis media with perforation and recurrent otorrhea complicated by nasopharyngeal obstruction and/or nasopharyngitis despite adequate medical therapy

D. Other
  1. Suspected malignancy of tonsillar or adenoidal tissue

II. Lab tests: (as indicated)

III. Other tests: (as indicated)

IV. Type of anesthesia: (as indicated)

V. Location of service: (as indicated)

---

*Clinical indicators for tonsil and adenoid surgery developed by the AAO HNS subcommittee here on quality assurance.

few patients should undergo adenoidectomy for these latter reasons alone, the few that should can benefit greatly.

Thus, most indications for adenoidectomy are philosophic. In prepubertal patients with recurrent streptococcal tonsillitis who are to be treated by tonsillectomy, adenoidectomy should usually be done at the same time. Encircling the oronasopharyngeal areas is a ring of lymphoid tissue known as Waldeyer's ring. The tonsils and the adenoids are the major lymphoid tissues of this ring. Most commonly, streptococcal tonsillitis involves the adenoids, and it is best to do an adenoidectomy concurrently with tonsillectomy. In patients with cleft palates and even in those with submucosal cleft palates in whom nasopharyngeal incompetence is at risk, adenoidectomy should be avoided; it is wise to avoid tonsillectomy as well.

Serous otitis media affects as many as 20% of school-age children. Its cause remains elusive and is most likely multifactorial. Clearly, in some patients, serous otitis media develops because of adenoidal obstruction of the eustachian tube at its entrance into the nasopharynx. These patients presumably will benefit by removal of the adenoids. No one knows what percentage of patients with prolonged serous otitis media associated with conductive hearing loss or retraction of the tympanic membrane have their eustachian tubes obstructed by adenoidal tissue. Therefore, patients with severe otitis media and large adenoids should be considered for adenoidectomy—carried out ordinarily at the time of myringotomy and insertion of ventilation tubes. Large adenoids are strongly suggested by nasal obstruction. However, once again, this is a philosophic decision that must be decided on mutually by the treating physician and the patient or the patient's parents. Similarly, if the patient has large tonsils, these may compress the inferior aspect of the eustachian tube, and tonsillectomy should be considered, particularly if the patient has a history of recurrent tonsillitis, and if the recurrent tonsillitis predisposes to ear infection.

The indications for T&A are summarized in Table 4.2. In 1988, the American Academy of Otolaryngology—Head and Neck Surgery (AAO HNS) developed its own clinical indicators for tonsil and adenoid surgery. These are reproduced in Table 4.3.

Morbidity and Mortality

Before an operation can be recommended, the physician must understand the risks that are incurred by such a procedure. The risks of morbidity and mortality from T&A range from postoperative throat discomfort to death.[5] In one of the largest studies of T&A, consisting of 6,175,729 cases, Pratt[6] showed a mortality of 1 in 16,381 (0.006%) (see Table 4.4). This study showed that anesthesia was responsible for 139 deaths, or 1 in 44,429 (0.002%). Cardiac arrest occurred in 27 patients, or 1 in 48,627 (0.002%). In the same study, hemorrhage was examined as a severe cause of morbidity. Catastrophic bleeding requiring carotid artery ligation occurred during the immediate post-

**Table 4.4 Morbidity and Mortality in 6,175,729
Tonsillectomies and Adenoidectomies***

CONDITION	%
Mortality	
Anesthesia	0.002
Cardiac arrest	0.002
Hemorrhage	0.002
Total	0.006
Hemorrhage	
Requiring carotid ligation	
Immediate postoperative period	0.008
Delayed postoperative period	0.020
Requiring 5 or more U of blood	0.009

*According to Pratt.[6]

operative period in 504 patients, that is, 1 in 12,253 (0.008%), and in the delayed postoperative period in 1496 patients, or 1 in 4128 (0.02%). Bleeding requiring transfusions of more than 5 U occurred in 538 patients, or 1 in 11,479 (0.009%). In 1965, Alexander[7] found the mortality rate to be 1.03 for every 10,000 tonsillectomies, with most deaths related to the following factors: (1) lack of observation, (2) use of ether anesthesia rather than halothane, (3) patients older than 15 years old, and (4) lack of decisiveness by the surgeon confronted with hemorrhage. No deaths occurred in patients in whom tonsillectomies were done under local anesthesia. Tolczynski[8] quoted the Commission for Professional Hospital Activities as finding that postoperative hemorrhage had the following incidence: ear, nose, and throat specialists, 1.9%; general surgeons, 2.5%; and general practitioners, 3.4%. One in 13 physicians in the study had at least one patient die because of bleeding following T&A.

Other complications of T&A procedures are numerous, including nasopharyngeal stenosis in approximately 3 in 100,000 T&As.[9,10] A variety of less common complications have been reported, including acute cervical adenitis, occasionally with abscess formation and suppuration,[11] extending to deep compartments of the neck; airway obstruction secondary to subglottic edema, resulting from intubation; aspiration of foreign bodies, particularly blood clots; mediastinal emphysema; rupture of pulmonary blebs and alveoli; otalgia; palatal incompetence; and food, fluids, and air escaping from the nose. Rhinolalia aperta (air escaping from the nose) is relatively common. However, it is uncommon for food, fluid, or air escaping from the nose to be a long-term sequela. Dental dislocation secondary to mouth gags and intubation occurs most frequently in children with deciduous teeth. Uvular edema often seen with cautery is common, but is rarely of significance. Uvular amputation can also occur but is of no significance.

A variety of diseases have been reported in association with tonsillectomy, including Hodgkin's disease,[12] multiple sclerosis,[13] and poliomyelitis.[14] None of these studies is definitive, although they seem conclusive; nevertheless, in almost all cases, there are additional studies equally well done that have differing conclusions. In all of these cases, it is difficult to screen out those patients in whom a disease (eg, Hodgkin's disease or appendicitis) would have developed despite the T&A. The indications used as the basis for carrying out T&A may represent the early manifestations of those diseases. Although it may be possible that the tonsils play an important role in protection against Hodgkin's disease, no one has ever provided strong evidence that this is true.[15]

The major causes of morbidity and mortality associated with these operations are as follows: All patients demonstrate the usual fears of surgical procedures, and almost all patients have a certain amount of postoperative discomfort. Postoperative bleeding may be as common as 1 in 100 cases, but it is seldom serious. Although it may be terrifying, it should result in death only rarely. Death from anesthesia also occurs. These causes, combined, result in a mortality of approximately 1 patient in 16,000 (0.006%).

Conclusions

The number of T&As carried out each year has been significantly reduced, yet many are still done without proper indications. Some patients who stand to benefit significantly from these procedures are denied the opportunity by physicians who are afraid of the risks posed by the operation or are unconvinced of its beneficial effects. Many surgeons who work with skilled anesthesiologists have few complications, and for these, indications can be broader. The converse is also true. Patients have fears, feelings, and philosophies. These, too, must be considered. Some patients need to be persuaded to have an operation and others must be dissuaded. This is the skill and art of medicine.

REFERENCES

1. Larsen JR, Bennett M. Adenotonsillectomy in children. *Wis Med J*. 1962; 61:561–567.
2. Ainger LE. Large tonsils and adenoids in small children with cor pulmonale. *Br Heart J*. 1968; 30:356–362.
3. Roydhouse N. A controlled study of adenotonsillectomy. *Lancet*. 1969; 2:931–932.
4. Paradise JL, Bluestone C. Toward rational indications for tonsil and adenoid surgery. *Hosp Pract* [Off]. 1976; 11:79–87.
5. Tate N. Deaths from tonsillectomy. *Lancet*. 1963; 7:1090–1091.
6. Pratt CW. Tonsillectomy and adenoidectomy: Mortality and morbidity. *Trans Am Acad Ophthalmol Otolaryngol*. 1970; 74:1146–1154.

7. Alexander D. Factors in tonsillectomy mortality. *Arch Otolaryngol*. 1965; 82:409–411.
8. Tolczynski B. Tonsillectomy, its hazards and their prevention. *Eye Ear Nose Throat Monthly*. 1969; 48:378–385.
9. Lehman WB. Nasopharyngeal stenosis. *Laryngoscope*. 1968; 78:371–385.
10. Imperatori CJ. Atresia of the pharynx operated upon by the Mackenty method. *Ann Otol Rhinol Laryngol*. 1944; 53:329–334.
11. Ritter FN. Tonsillectomy and adenoidectomy—Indications and complications. *Postgrad Med*. 1967; 41:342–347.
12. Vianna NJ, Greenwald P, Davies JNP. Tonsillectomy and Hodgkin's disease: The lymphoid tissue barrier. *Lancet*. 1971; L:431–432.
13. Poskanzer DC. Tonsillectomy and multiple sclerosis. *Lancet*. 1964; 2:1264–1265.
14. Aycock WL, Luther EH. Occurrence of poliomyelitis following tonsillectomy. *N Engl J Med* 1929; 200:167–167.
15. Davidson TM. Tonsillectomy and Hodgkin's disease. *Arch Otolaryngol Head Neck Surg*. 1973; 97:497.

CHAPTER 5

Neck Masses: Differential Diagnosis and Evaluation

Lumps in the neck are a frequent diagnostic dilemma. Clear thinking and proper evaluation will successfully uncover the diagnosis without causing the patient undue harm or cost. Neck masses can be divided into five broad etiologic categories: congenital, traumatic, inflammatory, neoplastic, and metabolic. Figures 5.1 and 5.2 are algorithms for the differential diagnosis of neck masses.

NECK MASSES RESULTING FROM CONGENITAL LESIONS

Congenital lesions are not always present at birth and can appear from birth to 30 years of age. Preauricular pits arise from the first branchial cleft and are the most common branchial cleft anomaly. Generally they give rise to a small sinus tract and are easily excised. Occasionally, they form a fistulous tract that communicates from the preauricular skin to the external auditory canal or to the nasopharynx. These fistulae can be intricately related to the facial nerve. Surgical excision must be done carefully to protect the peripheral branches of the facial nerve.

Branchial cleft cysts and sinuses result from developmental errors. However, they do not present until they fill with fluid, become infected, or drain through a cutaneous sinus or fistula. The second branchial cleft cyst presents as a swelling in the neck, and it may become infected. Usually, it lies anterior to the sternocleidomastoid muscle at the level of the hyoid bone. Its embryonic connection is to the ipsilateral tonsil. This is generally difficult to see. At least theoretically, third and fourth branchial cleft cysts may also form. If they occur, they would present similarly but would connect to the piriform sinus or esophagus, respectively. These cysts may present at any age, but they seem to be most common during the 20s and 30s. If they first appear as a swelling without infection, they can be removed at a patient's convenience, but they should be excised because they are

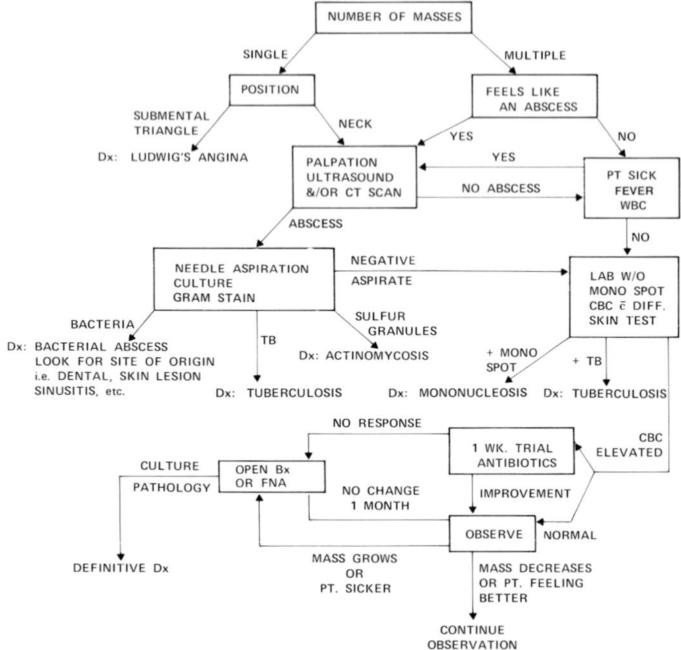

Figure 5.1. Algorithm for differential diagnosis of inflammatory neck mass. Dx = diagnosis; CT = computed tomography; CBC = complete blood cell count; PT = patient; Bx = biopsy; WBC = white neck mass. Dx = diagnosis; CT = computed tomography; CBC = complete blood cell count; PT = patient, Bx = biopsy; WBC = white blood cell count.

at risk for infection. A cyst presented as an infected mass should be treated with antibiotics. If the infection can be cleared medically, surgery to remove the cyst and prevent further infection should be performed 3 to 5 weeks later. If however, the cyst develops into an abscess, excision and drainage are necessary. This is a difficult procedure and must be done under general anesthesia by a skilled surgeon. The cyst may then be removed 3 to 6 weeks later.

Thyroglossal duct cysts occur in the midline anywhere from the hyoid bone to the suprasternal notch. They can appear as a swelling, or, like the branchial cleft cyst, as an infection. The infection must be treated appropriately and the cyst with its sinus tract excised. The sinus tract communicates from the cyst to the foramen cecum at the base of the tongue. It courses around the hyoid bone, and the middle third of the hyoid must be removed at surgery or the cyst will recur.

Hemangiomas and lymphangiomas occur most commonly in the

head and neck. Although many are pure hemangiomas or lymphangiomas, some are combinations. They tend to present in the first several years after birth and may be noticed in the oral cavity, in the neck, or on the face. They are easy to diagnose because they are soft and diffuse. They do not have well-defined borders. A massive lymphangioma of the neck is called a cystic hygroma. Generally, these tumors proliferate, sometimes rapidly and extensively during early childhood, but all will regress eventually. Surgery is difficult and often dangerous to adjacent structures. Surgery is indicated only to preserve the airway or for extensive tumors affecting multiple head and neck structures. Residual lesions are often removed during the teens and early 20s for cosmetic reasons. Hemangiomas involving the skin are treated similarly.

NECK MASSES RESULTING FROM TRAUMA

Traumatic lesions presenting as a neck mass are uncommon. Generally, the physician and the patient easily associate the neck mass with the trauma. Most gunshot wounds and stabbing wounds of the neck should be explored surgically and damaged structures repaired. A traumatic vascular injury can cause an arteriovenous fistula, which will present as a pulsatile mass with an audible bruit. Arteriography confirms the diagnosis. Surgical ligation is indicated.

A laryngocele is a diverticulum arising from the laryngeal ventricle, usually on the left side. It usually presents in the neck as a soft tissue mass that comes and goes. It is most commonly found in musicians playing wind instruments, such as the tuba or trumpet. The mass inflates while playing and deflates when the pressure is relived. A CT scan or a contrast laryngogram may confirm the diagnosis. Because laryngoceles continue to grow with time and because they have a potential for infection, they are usually removed surgically.

The esophagus can also develop a pulsion diverticulum. This is called a Zenker's diverticulum and presents as a mass in the left side of the neck. It arises from the posterior wall of the esophagus just above the superior esophageal sphincter. Symptoms usually include a history of regurgitating food. The food may be regurgitated hours after eating, and unlike the situation with gastric regurgitation, the food is not digested. Patients may also complain of swallowing difficulty (dysphagia). Barium swallow and esophagoscopy are diagnostic. Infection is rare. Surgery is indicated for symptomatic lesions.

NECK MASSES RESULTING FROM INFLAMMATORY LESIONS

Inflammatory lesions are the most common cause of neck masses, especially in children and young adults.

Viral lymphadenitis is universal in children with viral upper RTIs. The swollen lymph nodes are multiple, soft, mobile, and rarely larger

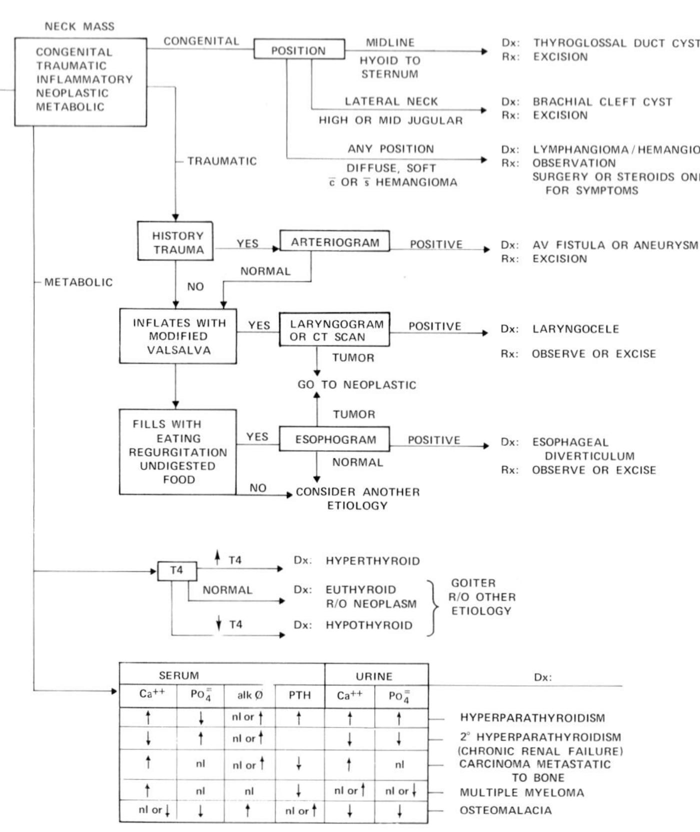

SERUM				URINE		Dx:
Ca^{++}	$PO_4^=$	alk Ø	PTH	Ca^{++}	$PO_4^=$	
↑	↓	nl or ↑	↑	↑	↑	HYPERPARATHYROIDISM
↓	↑	nl or ↑		↓	↓	2° HYPERPARATHYROIDISM (CHRONIC RENAL FAILURE)
↑	nl	nl or ↑	↓	↑	nl	CARCINOMA METASTATIC TO BONE
↑	nl	nl	↓	nl or ↑	nl or ↓	MULTIPLE MYELOMA
nl or ↓	↓	↑	nl or ↑	↓	↓	OSTEOMALACIA

Figure 5.2.   Algorithm for differential diagnosis of neoplastic neck mass. Dx = diagnosis; Bx = biopsy; R/O = rule out. *(Continued on p. 133.)*

than 2-cm across. Occasionally, one will grow significantly larger. The clinician must then decide if this is simply a large node or if it has become infected and abscessed. Mumps and some other viruses infect the parotid and occasionally the submandibular salivary glands. The clinical history, the bilaterality, and the position of the masses should help make the diagnosis of sialoadenitus.

Bacterial abscess is a common problem in the neck. It may complicate either a viral or a bacterial upper respiratory tract infection. This can originate from the skin, the ear, the nose, the paranasal sinuses, the oral cavity, especially the teeth, the oropharynx, or a traumatic injury to the mucosa or skin. There can be a solitary abscess

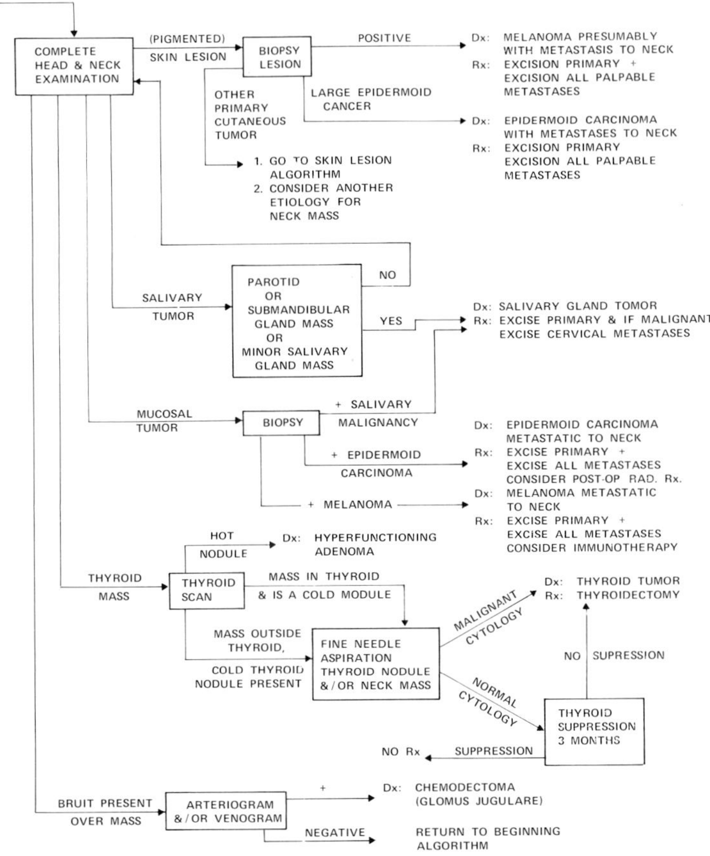

Figure 5.2. (continued)

or multiple matted, infected, and abscessed nodes. Patients with an abscess may be sick and extremely toxic. The mass can be firm, if it is under pressure, or it may feel fluctuant. Aspiration of pus is diagnostic. Ultrasound can help differentiate soft tissue swelling from a fluid- or pus-filled mass. Most cervical abscesses contain mixed anaerobic organisms. Diagnosis and treatment of a neck abscess is complex because the neck contains several different potential spaces wherein an abscess can form. These involve the perispinal space, the perivisceral spaces, or the perivascular spaces. Surgical drainage is mandatory and must be done by a skilled head and neck surgeon under general anesthesia.

If the patient has risk factors for AIDS, then one of the lympho-proliferative disorders must be considered. Single or multiple neck masses, large or small can be the first clinical sign of AIDS. The work-up should include a complete blood count and human immu-nodeficiency virus (HIV) serology. Skin testing for tuberculosis and fungal disease is indicated. An open biopsy is ultimately required. For the AIDS patient, this distinguishes between lymphoid hyperpla-sia, lymphoma, and metastatic cancer. The most important point is that AIDS can present as a cervical neck mass. If surgery is required, the precautions listed in the section on AIDS are mandatory.

A variety of other infectious agents may cause a cervical mass. Tuberculosis is common and may be confined to the neck. Diagnosis is sometimes difficult. The patient undergoes skin tests, and material is submitted for staining and culturing. Medical therapy is usually curative. Coccidioidomycosis can present in the neck, but rarely with-out florid pulmonary involvement. Mycobacteria and atypical my-cobacteria can also cause infections that present as cervical disease. Most fungal infections can be identified by specific skin tests. Fresh tissue can be submitted for culture. Actinomycosis usually presents as a neck mass that drains from the oral cavity to the skin. Typical sulfur granules will make the histologic diagnosis. If sulfur granules are not found, cultures are easily grown. Syphilis and cat-scratch fever can also present as neck masses. Both must be suspected from the history. Diagnosis of syphilis is serologic, and cat-scratch fever is recognized by the clinical picture and by biopsy. A variety of other infectious diseases can involve cervical lymph nodes. Generally they will produce symptoms that are more evident elsewhere in the body, but occasionally, the cervical biopsy and culture will be diagnostic. Mononucleosis may also involve the neck. In this condition, nodes are large, soft, and multiple. The diagnosis is made clinically and serologically.

Diagnosis of Infectious Neck Masses

The general work-up for a presumably infectious neck mass can be complex. An acute abscess must be evaluated on an emergent basis. The patient is admitted to the hospital, and appropriate examinations and consultations are obtained immediately. If the patient is ill but the mass is not abscessed, sample material from needle aspiration is sent for culture, sensitivity tests, and Gram stain. The patient is placed on a regimen of penicillin, 10 to 20 million U IV daily. O IV antibiotic regimens may be used. If the patient remains toxic, surgery is nec-essary. If the patient is not acutely ill, appropriate skin tests and serologic tests are ordered and evaluated. A trial of antibiotics is often used. If no diagnosis is made and the mass continues to grow, ex-ploration, excision, or biopsy is undertaken, and sample material is submitted for culture and pathologic examination. Certainly a consultation with an infectious disease specialist and a head and neck surgeon should be requested for all these patients.

Ludwig's angina is an abscess involving the floor of the mouth. It is described here because it is potentially life-threatening if not treated appropriately. Patients present with fever and mild toxicity early in the disease. They become increasingly toxic as the abscess progresses. There is usually swelling and tenderness under the chin, with little intraoral evidence of the disease. As the abscess enlarges, which it can do rapidly, the tongue is forced back in the mouth. The airway becomes rapidly obstructed. All patients with this condition should be brought to the operating room and the abscess drained under general anesthesia. Intravenous antibiotic therapy is also begun immediately. Formerly, many patients required tracheostomy, but as physician awareness has increased, the diagnosis is being made earlier and tracheostomy is required less frequently.

NECK MASSES RESULTING FROM NEOPLASTIC LESIONS

Neoplasms may present in the neck. Several types of neoplasms are common.

Lymphoma may present in early and middle adulthood. The masses are usually multiple and can be bilateral or unilateral. They can be as small as 1 to 2 cm or as large as 6 to 10 cm. They are soft and mobile. Lymphomas may involve the posterior or anterior triangles of the neck. Other lymphoid tissue, such as the tonsils, may also be involved. The patient may be otherwise asymptomatic or may have low-grade fever, malaise, and occasionally some weight loss. Diagnosis is made by biopsy and histologic evaluation.

Epidermoid carcinoma is a tumor found in middle and late adulthood. It is strongly associated with tobacco use. The carcinogenic effect of the tobacco is enhanced by alcohol. The primary tumor will be found on one of the mucosal surfaces of the upper respiratory–digestive tract. The neck disease is metastatic. The neck mass can be unilateral or bilateral, single or multiple. The mass feels hard to palpation and can be fixed due to invasion of adjoining structures. Patients often show weight loss: fever and malaise are not common. Diagnosis should be made by discovering the primary lesion and taking a biopsy specimen. The primary tumor and the cervical metastasis are treated as an entity. To perform biopsy on the neck without discovering the primary tumor can seriously jeopardize the final cure.

Tumors of the chest and abdomen can metastasize to the neck via the thoracic duct. These metastases are palpable masses just above the clavicle in the supraclavicular fossa. The thoracic duct joins the jugular or subclavian veins near their junction in the supraclavicular fossa. Although the left side is most commonly involved, right-sided lesions are also found from right-sided or accessory thoracic ducts.

These tumors do not usually present as masses higher in the neck. Although a full head and neck examination is recommended, lymph node biopsy should be performed early to direct the search for the primary lesion.

Thyroid tumors and their cervical metastases will usually present as an asymptomatic neck mass. The thyroid lies low in the anterior neck and, of course, moves up and down with swallowing. Work-up should include thyroid scan and ultrasonography. Cold nodules are diagnosed by biopsy. The diagnosis of a cervical metastasis from a small thyroid mass will usually not be obvious until the histologic nature of the neck mass is determined.

A variety of other tumors, such as melanoma, sarcoma, plasmacytoma, and adenocarcinoma, may all present as neck masses. Diagnosis is made by a full work-up and a biopsy.

Fine needle aspiration plays an increasingly important role in the evaluation of cervical disease. A clinic procedure with minimal risk, FNA is useful for inflammatory (especially infectious) lesions and neoplastic tumors.

The site to be biopsied is cleaned with povidone-iodine or with alcohol. One percent lidocaine with 1/100,000 epinephrine is injected into the skin. A 22-gauge needle is placed on a 10- or 20-cc syringe and held in an aspirator as shown in Figure 5.3. The needle is inserted into the mass and the plunger pulled back to create a negative pressure. If an inflammatory lesion is encountered, infected fluid will be aspirated, which will be tested for appropriate cultures including bacteria, tuberculosis, and fungi. If a solid lesion is encountered, the negative pressure is maintained while the needle is moved back and forth in the mass. Effectively, the needle cuts off cells from the tumor that are then captured in the needle. After three or four passes, the needle is removed and the cellular material injected onto a slide. The

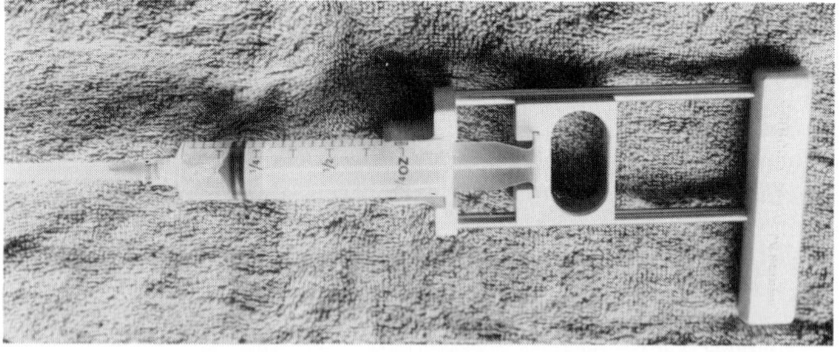

Figure 5.3.   A 20-cc syringe in a holder used for fine needle aspiration. The syringe holder permits the physician to hold the negative pressure necessary to perform the aspiration with high vacuum.

material is smeared across the slide and then prepared for cytologic evaluation.

Fine needle aspiration cytology is useful in diagnosing malignancy. It is most useful in the head and neck for diagnosis of salivary gland tumors, thyroid tumors, and metastatic epidermoid carcinoma. It is generally not adequate for lymphoproliferative disorders. Although a positive FNA is very useful, a negative FNA does not exclude a neoplasm, and generally one must then proceed to an open biopsy.

NECK MASSES RESULTING FROM METABOLIC DISORDERS

Metabolic disease involving the thyroid or parathyroid glands can present as a neck mass. Hyperthyroidism should have obvious clinical manifestations and be readily diagnosable with tests for tetra iodothyronine (T_4), tri-iodothyronine (T_3), thyroid-stimulating hormone (TSH), and thyroid uptake, as well as a thyroid scan. A goiter can present in an otherwise asymptomatic person. The mass is obvious on physical exam. Thyroid work-up and scan should be diagnostic. Biopsy is rarely needed. Parathyroid tumors may be asymptomatic and in this case will be difficult to differentiate from a cold thyroid nodule. Parathyroid adenomas will present with hypercalcemia.

In closing this chapter, several case histories are presented to highlight and illustrate this information. (Case Studies A–D).

Case Study A

A 28-year-old woman presented with a progressively enlarging mass in her left neck (Fig. 5.4). It was painful and it hurt to open her mouth or chew. Past medical history and review of systems were noncontributory.

Physical Examination

Temperature: 101.5°F orally.
Skin: red and edematous over mass.
Eyes, PERRL, EOM WNL, fundi clear.
Ears: Weber midline; Rinne AC > BC AU (256 cps).
Nose: normal.
Mouth: Patient has trismus. Swelling is present over left mandibular molar, which is chipped.
Neck: 5–6-cm tender mass present under the left mandible—or mass is firm.

Differential Diagnosis

Congenital lesions: Second branchial cleft cyst (unlikely).
Trauma: no history.

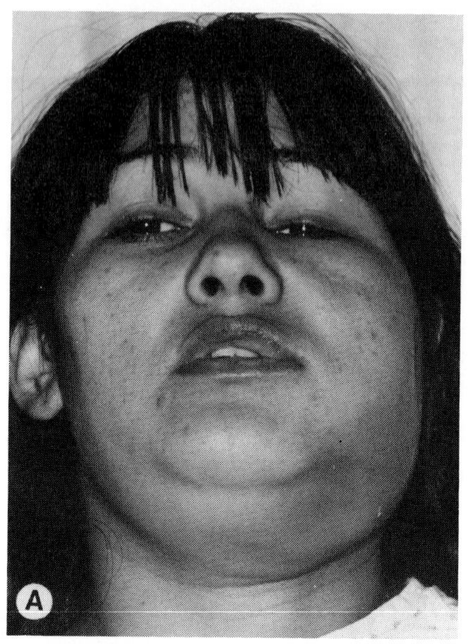

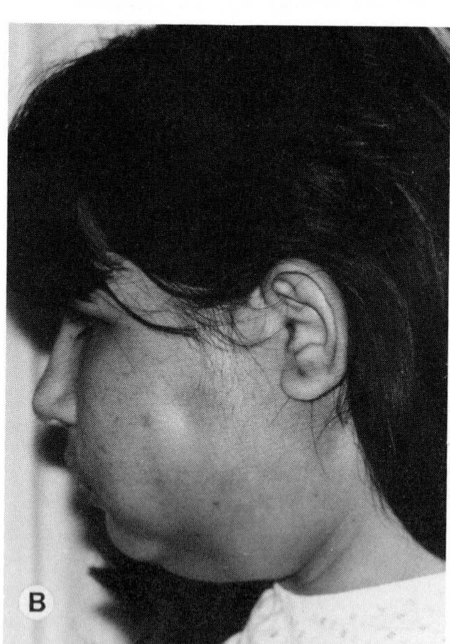

Figure 5.4.   Two views of a patient with a neck mass.

Inflammatory: Abscess secondary to dental infection. Tuberculosis or atypical mycobacteria infection.
Neoplasms: Always must be excluded.
Metabolic: No history of endocrine problems.

A dental consultation was obtained, and an X ray (Fig. 5.5) was taken. This shows a fractured second molar tooth and a periapical abscess. The patient was hospitalized and therapy was begun with 2.4 million U of IV penicillin q4h. The next day the tooth was extracted and pus was drained from the socket. Unfortunately, the neck mass progressed in size and became fluctuant. The patient was brought to the operating room, and under general anesthesia, a submandibular space abscess was incised and drained. Several species of anaerobes were cultured. Defervescence occurred and the patient recovered rapidly.

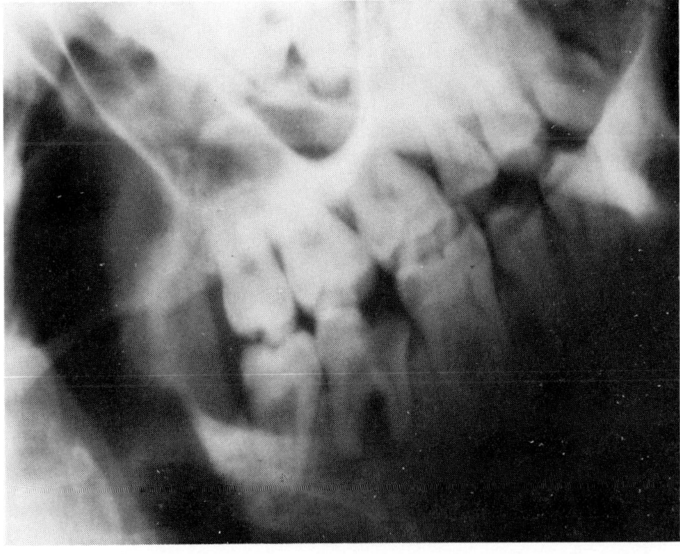

Figure 5.5. X ray of dental infection. Note the fractured second molar and the periapical abscess seen as a lucent area surrounding the second molar tooth roots.

Case Study B

An 18-year-old white male presented with the chief complaint of a "lump" in his neck of 1-week's duration. The patient had been well until 3 weeks previously, when he developed a sore throat. This persisted 2 days and then progressed into a purulent runny nose. This was treated with decongestants and aspirin. The rhinorrhea resolved over the subsequent 7 days, but then the patient discovered a lump in the left side of his neck. This lump remained unchanged for 1 week, during which time the patient ran a low-grade fever and had some mild malaise, but showed no weight loss. The past medical history and review of systems were noncontributory. The patient denied previous, recent, or old trauma. He did not have any unusual infectious diseases and no known history of neck irradiation. His family history was unknown and unobtainable.

On examination, his blood pressure was 120/80, pulse rate 75, respirations 20, and temperature 99.1°F.

Physical Examination

Skin: clear with a few facial comedones.
Eyes: PERRLA, EOM WNL. Fundi clear.
Ears: hearing normal to tuning forks. TMs gray and translucent with normal movement to pneumomassage.
Nose: mucosa red and the septum deviated to the left.
Mouth: normal; dentition good, without caries or fillings.
Nasopharynx: poorly visualized by mirror examination.
Larynx: well seen and entirely normal.
Neck: there is a 2 × 3 cm smooth, soft but not fluctuant, mobile mass in the mid-left neck overlying the jugular vein. Multiple other shotty nodes are palpable along both jugular veins.
The remainder of the physical examination was normal.

Differential Diagnosis

Congenital lesions: Second branchial cleft cyst.
Trauma: No history.
Inflammatory: Residual viral adenopathy. Bacterial abscess in a cervical lymph node secondary to upper respiratory tract infection. Tuberculosis or atypical mycobacterium. Cat scratch fever. Fungal disease.
Neoplasm: rule out lymphoma or other uncommon neoplasm.
Metabolic: no history of endocrine problems.

Laboratory Data

CBC:
Hgb—13
Hct—9

WBC—8500
   Segs—54
   Lymphs—40 with no atypicals
   Monos—4
   Eosinophils—2
Sed rate: 12
Skin Test: TB, histo, cocci, mumps all negative.

Chest X ray: Normal, no evidence of any pulmonary disease.
Ultrasound of the neck shows a relatively homogeneous soft
   tissue mass. No cystic spaces identified.

Discussion

Most likely this was an inflammatory lesion, but lymphoma
had to be excluded. The mass had not changed significantly for
3 weeks, and so the patient was brought to the operating room.
Under general anesthesia the nasopharynx and larynx were examined directly. No abnormalities were seen. The neck was
explored and the entire lymph node excised. The specimen was
brought fresh to the pathologist. Pieces were sent for aerobic
and anaerobic bacterial cultures, *mycobacterium tuberculosis*
cultures, atypical mycobacterium cultures, and fungal cultures.
Touch preparations were made, a piece of tissue was set aside
for electron microscopy, and the remainder of the tissue was
fixed in formalin. The impression gained from permanent sections was of an inflammatory lesion with granulomatous reactions. Tuberculosis was not demonstrated by special stains.
There was no evidence of lymphoma. A presumptive diagnosis
of cervical tuberculosis was made. A specialist in pulmonary
medicine was consulted and a regimen of antituberculosis medication was instituted. Six weeks later the cultures for tuberculosis finally became positive.

Case Study C

A 45-year-old businessman presented with a chief complaint
of a lump in his neck of 1-week's duration. The patient first
noticed this while shaving. He had been in good health, without
any recent diseases. He noted a 10-lb weight loss, but believed
this was due to his recent efforts to diet. The patient had smoked
two packs of cigarettes daily for 25 years, and drank two to
three cocktails daily. He had an American lifestyle, but was
born and lived in Japan until the age of 15 years. He did not
know much about his medical past. Current past medical history
and review of systems were noncontributory.

Examination revealed a worried but otherwise healthy Japanese male about 20 pounds overweight. Blood pressure was 140/90, pulse 85, respirations 22, temperature 98.6°F.

Physical Examination

Skin: normal and without any lesions.
Eyes: PERRLA EOM WNL. Fundi show mild vascular changes.
Ears: Weber—midline. Rinne AC > BC AU.
Nose: red mucosa, septum deviated to left.
Mouth: teeth in poor repair. No mucosal lesions seen.
Nasopharynx: poorly visualized by mirror exam.
Larynx: well seen. Vocal cords move normally, but both hyperemic.
Neck: a 2 × 3 cm firm mobile nontender mass is present in the left midjugular region.
The remainder of the exam was noncontributory.

Differential Diagnosis

Congenital lesions: very unlikely.
Trauma: no history for traumatic injury.
Inflammatory: rule out tuberculosis, coccidomycossis, atypical mycobacterium.
Neoplastic (most likely) epidermoid cancer metastatic from upper aerodigestive tract. Rule our thyroid tumor: metastatic. Lymphoma.
Metabolic: no history of endocrine abnormality.

Laboratory Data

CBC:
  Hct—39
  Hgb—13
  WBC 6500
Urinalysis: normal
Creatinine: 1.2
Bilirubin, alkaline phosphatase normal.
Chest X ray: mild COPD. No evidence of TB or tumor.
Thyroid scan: normal.
Sinus series: normal.
Skin tests: TB, histo, cocci all negative. Mumps positive.
FNA: epidermoid carcinoma

Discussion

The patient was brought to the operating room and under general anesthesia nasopharyngoscopy, laryngoscopy, bronchoscopy, and esophagoscopy were performed. No significant abnormalities were revealed. Because of the high risk for an epidermoid neoplasm, random biopsy specimens were taken from the nasopharynx, base of the tongue, and piriform sinuses. These are areas known to hide occult neoplasms. Frozen section of a specimen from the left nasopharyngeal eustachian tube orifice revealed a moderately differentiated epidermoid cancer. After the patient was awakened, the nasopharynx and neck were treated with radical radiation therapy.

Had the FNA and the mucosal biopsies failed to find any lesion, an open biopsy would have been performed. The specimen would have been brought fresh to the pathologist for cultures for bacteria, *Mycobacterium tuberculosis,* atypical mycobacterium, and fungi; for frozen section; for touch preparations; and for permanent pathologic specimens. A piece would have been saved for electron microscopy. The frozen section would have shown epidermoid cancer and a standard lymph node dissection would have been performed. Postoperative irradiation would have been used depending on final pathology reports and the viewpoints about treatment of both the treating physicians and the patient. However, proper evaluations correctly identified the primary tumor, saved the patient from unnecessary surgery, and improved his chance of cure.

Case Study D

A 22-year-old housewife presented with a chief complaint of a lump in her neck of 1-week's duration. The patient was in good health and first noticed this lump 1 week earlier after showering. She denied having any recent diseases. She had smoked one-half pack of cigarettes per day for the past 7 years and did not drink alcohol. She had no history of radiation therapy as a child. She had no fever and malaise, but had noted a 10-lb weight loss over the past 2 months, which she attributed to her dieting. Her past medical history and review of symptoms were noncontributory. Her only positive finding on history was a mole removed from behind her left ear 1 year earlier. Pathologic examination showed this to be benign.

Physical Examination

Blood Pressure: 120/75.
Pulse 68, respirations 16.
Temperature: 98.5°F.
Skin: well healed scar behind left ear.
Eyes: PERRLA EOM WNL. Fundi benign.
Ears: Weber: midline Rinne: AC > BC AU (256 cps). TMs
   gray, translucent, normal mobility.
Nose: red mucosa; septum straight.

Mouth: normal.
Nasopharynx: well seen, without lesions.
Larynx: well seen, normal.
Neck: 2 × 3 cm midjugular node, firm and mobile; 1 × 1 cm node, high jugular; 1 × 2 cm node, low jugular—all left side.
The remainder of the physical examination was noncontributory.

Differential Diagnosis

Congenital: multiple nodes exclude this diagnosis.
Trauma: multiple nodes exclude this diagnosis.
Inflammatory: rule out TB, atypical mycobacterium, fungal infection, or benign adenopathy secondary to head and neck infection.
Neoplastic: epidermoid cancer unlikely. Thyroid cancer unlikely but rule out other tumors (all unlikely).
Metabolic: no history of endocrine disease.

Laboratory Data

CBC:
  Hct—39
  Hgb—13
WBC—8500 with normal differential
Urinalysis: normal
Creatinine: 0.8
Bilirubin, alkaline phosphatase: normal.
Chest X ray: normal.
Thyroid scan with technetium shows three masses in the neck with increased uptake. The thyroid gland is normal.
Sinus series: mucosal thickening in the left maxillary sinus.
Skin tests: TB, histo, cocci, mumps all negative.
FNA: Nondiagnostic; malignant cells suspected.

Discussion

The patient was placed on antibiotic therapy for 2 weeks, during which time no change in the masses occurred. She was then brought to the operating room and triple endoscopy was performed. No suspicious lesions were seen, and no random biopsy samples were taken. The 2 × 3 cm mass was excised and brought fresh to the pathologist. Pieces were sent for culture for bacteria (both aerobic and anaerobic), *Mycobacterium tuberculosis,* atypical mycobacteria, and fungi. Additional pieces were processed for permanent section and frozen section, and a piece saved for electron microscopy. Frozen section showed a malignancy, type unknown. The incision was closed. Permanent section likewise did not reveal the type of malignancy. Old slides from the previous skin tumor were obtained. No diagnosis could be made and the original block specimen was requested. Electron microscopy showed that the cervical mass was a melanoma. Recutting the original skin lesion specimen showed that this indeed was the primary site. The patient underwent lymph node dissection and then radical radiation therapy.

CHAPTER 6

Head and Neck Cancer

In 1990, the American Cancer Society reported 1,740,000 new malignancies. There were 600,000 nonmelanoma skin cancers (primarily basal cell and squamous cell tumors). During the same 1-year period, 27,600 new melanomas were reported. Also during the same period, 61,400 new head and neck cancers were reported. This is 5% of all new noncutaneous malignant cancers. Ninety percent of the nonmelanoma skin cancers involved the head and neck.

Many different tumors are seen in the head and neck region; for purposes of discussion, each major type will be discussed separately.

EPIDERMOID CANCER

The most common tumor of the head and neck region is epidermoid cancer arising on the mucosal surfaces of the upper aerodigestive tract. These tumors clearly are induced by tobacco carcinogens, whose effect is greatly enhanced by use of alcohol. Patients generally have a long history of tobacco use, such as having smoked two packs of cigarettes daily for 25 years. These tumors usually are not seen until the fourth decade of life. Generally, they begin as areas of dysplasia that develop into carcinoma in situ. When these tumors transgress the basement membrane and invade the underlying stroma, they are called invasive. The lymphatics of the submucosa are rich and regional metastasis to the cervical lymph nodes is common, particularly with advanced tumors. Distant metastasis tends to occur late.

The most common local symptoms are pain, voice changes, difficulty in breathing, difficulty in swallowing, weight loss, and malaise. The tumors are classified by sites in the head and neck. These sites include: the nasal cavity and paranasal sinuses; nasopharynx; oral cavity, which includes the lip; oropharynx; hypopharynx; and the larynx and cervical esophagus. The tumors are classified by the TNM staging system. In this system, the T stands for tumor, which is classified by size or by degree of extension. For example, in the oral cavity T_{IS} is carcinoma in situ, T_1 is an invasive tumor less than 2 cm in diameter, T_2 cancer is 2 to 4 cm in diameter, T_3 is greater than 4 cm, and T_4 is massive tumor invading bone or extending beyond the oral cavity. The N stands for regional lymph node involvement. N_0 refers to no clinically positive nodes; N_1 is a single ipsilateral node (ie, on the same side as the tumor) less than 3 cm in diameter. N_2 is a single ipsilateral node 3 to 6 cm in diameter or multiple ipsilateral nodes all less than 6 cm in diameter. N_3 is a single ipsilateral node greater than 6 cm or a contralateral node or nodes, or bilateral nodes. M refers to metastases; M_0 means no known distant metastases and M_1 means distant metastases are present. The TNM is a clinical staging system based on the physical examination and laboratory data; tumors discovered by pathologic examination or by surgical exploration are not included. The classifications are complex, and most physicians have TNM staging summaries available for quick consultation.

Case Study: Epidermoid Cancer 1

A 56-year-old retired marine captain complained to his dentist that his mouth was sore. On examination the dentist detected a hard, ulcerated lesion on the tip of the tongue. The patient was referred to a head and neck surgeon. The sore had been present for 2 months. The patient had smoked two packs of cigarettes every day for 35 years and had imbibed a pint of whisky daily for the past 20 years. He had noted no weight loss. Physical examination revealed a 1.5-cm firm, ulcerated, tender lesion on the tip of the tongue. The remainder of the head and neck examination was normal. No masses were palpable in the neck. The patient was admitted to the hospital. A full laboratory evaluation revealed slightly elevated serum glutamic-pyruvic transaminase levels, believed to be due to the patient's history of alcohol intake. Chest X ray showed chronic pulmonary changes, but no suspicious lesions.

The patient was given general anesthesia and nasopharyngoscopy, laryngoscopy, esophagoscopy, and bronchoscopy with washings revealed no other tumors. The oral cavity lesion was biopsied and the histologic diagnosis was a well-differentiated epidermoid cancer. The patient was presented to the Combined Head and Neck Oncology Conference. He was believed to have a $T_1N_0M_0$ epidermoid cancer of the oral cavity. Surgery and radiation were believed to have equal cure rates. Surgery was chosen because it would cause very little deficit. Radiation would have required 5 to 7 weeks of therapy and would have left the patient with a dry mouth and long-term dental problems.

Diagnosis

All patients are evaluated with a complete history and physical examination. Laboratory data obtained include complete blood cell count, urinalysis, determinations of creatinine, blood urea nitrogen, alkaline phosphatase, and bilirubin (total and direct) levels. All patients have a chest X ray. Patients with head and neck tumors have at least a 10% incidence of second primary neoplasms, and a large fraction of these are pulmonary. Additional laboratory data, such as radioactive isotope scans, have not been helpful for staging or detecting metastatic disease. CT scan and MRI help to assess the extent of tumor in the primary site and neck. Metastatic disease tends to remain microscopic and has been difficult to detect clinically.

Nasopharyngoscopy, laryngoscopy, esophagoscopy, and bronchoscopy are all performed under general anesthesia. The primary tumor is biopsied. The patient is then evaluated at a combined conference of surgeons, radiation therapists, and medical oncologists. A treatment plan is recommended to the patient.

Case Study: Epidermoid Cancer 2

A 52-year-old nursery school teacher presented to her family doctor complaining of hoarseness of 2 weeks' duration. The physician examined her throat and told her she had laryngitis. He prescribed penicillin for 1 week. Initially the hoarseness improved, but then it rapidly returned. The patient went back to her physician, who referred her to a head and neck surgeon. She had smoked one and a half pack of cigarettes daily for 30 years. She did not drink alcohol. She had noted a 5-lb weight loss over the preceding month. Head and neck examination revealed a whitish, raised growth along the right vocal cord. The remainder of the head and neck examination was normal. The patient was admitted to the hospital. Laboratory and X-ray evaluations were all normal. The patient was anesthetized and endoscopic examinations performed. Laryngoscopy confirmed a lesion confined to the right true vocal cord. A biopsy specimen was taken. Histologic diagnosis was a well-differentiated epidermoid cancer.

The patient was presented to the Combined Head and Neck Oncology Conference. She was believed to have a $T_1N_0M_0$ epidermoid carcinoma of the larynx. Surgery would require a partial laryngectomy, which is a significant surgical undertaking, and the patient would have had problems postoperatively with aspiration and would never regain a normal voice. Radiation would require 7 weeks of treatment, but it could be done on an outpatient basis and would not create any major disability. Radiation therapy was recommended.

Treatment

Small lesions whose eradication by surgical means would not be disabling or disfiguring are treated by surgery. Small tumors for which surgery would be disabling are best treated by radiation therapy. Large tumors or any tumor associated with lymph nodes greater than 2 cm should be treated initially with surgery and then followed with radiation therapy. Chemotherapy is only an adjunctive or palliative treatment.

Case Study: Epidermoid Cancer 3

A 62-year-old male was brought to the hospital because he was coughing up blood. He had lost 30 lb over the past 3 months. He had smoked one pack of unfiltered cigarettes daily for 40 years and was what he described as a "social" drinker. The remainder of the patient's medical history was noncontributory. The medical work-up was extensive and was directed toward a pulmonary neoplasm. Chest X ray and CT scan did not discover any pathologic lesion. Fiberoptic bronchoscopy also failed to discover any significant abnormality. One sputum sample sent for cytologic study was read as Class V, showing frankly malignant cells. As part of the regular work-up for hemoptysis, a head and neck surgery consultation was requested. Mirror laryngeal examination discovered an abnormality behind the larynx. This area is called the postcricoid region, is part of the hypopharynx, and is very difficult to visualize. Neck examination revealed a 4-cm lymph node in the midjugular area and a 2-cm node just beneath it, both on the left side. Barium swallow with cine examination of the cervical esophagus showed a 4-cm, irregular mass in the hypopharynx. The patient was brought to the operating room. Bronchoscopy, laryngoscopy, and esophagoscopy were performed. A 4-cm tumor involving the posterior larynx and the entire entrance to the cervical esophagus was seen and biopsied. Pathologic diagnosis was a poorly differentiated epidermoid cancer.

The patient was presented to the Combined Head and Neck Oncology Conference. The tumor was classified as a $T_3N_2M_0$ epidermoid cancer of the hypopharynx. Members of the head and neck surgery team recommended a laryngopharyngectomy, a left neck lymph node dissection, and reconstruction of the esophagus with a pectoralis myocutaneous flap. This would be followed by postoperative radiation therapy. The radiation therapists suggested that the radiation be given preoperatively because if there were any problems with the esophageal reconstruction, postoperative radiation would be delayed, and this would compromise the patient's chance of cure. The surgeons pointed out that surgery following radiation therapy had a 30%

to 50% rate of wound infection because of the damage to the blood supply following irradiation. Wound infection rates for the same surgery prior to radiation therapy were 5% to 10%. The advantages and disadvantages of the two treatment plans were debated. It was decided that both treatment plans would be presented to the patient, and he and his wife would make their own decision about treatment.

Prognosis

The overall cure rate is about 60% for epidermoid head and neck cancers. Early lesions without cervical metastasis may be cured in 90% of cases, whereas large, advanced tumors with cervical metastasis have cure rates as low as 15% or 20%. Optimally, prevention would be possible by decreasing or eliminating tobacco use, but this is not occurring rapidly in the United States. The next most important measure would be to make people aware of the early signs of cancer and to encourage them to bring problems to their physician's attention as soon as possible. Finally, physicians and dentists must always be sensitive to the signs of head and neck malignancy. Patients at serious risk must be carefully examined early.

Problems with Difficult Diagnoses

It is always difficult to know exactly when a patient with a sore throat or similar symptom should be referred to a head and neck surgeon and when the condition can be treated by a primary care physician not skilled in the complete head and neck examination. The following case study should put this in some perspective.

Case Study: Epidermoid Cancer 4

The patient presented to the University Hospital with a 1-year history of a sore throat, which had been treated by his personal physician. On examination, a tumor was easily seen in the epiglottis. This was biopsied, and the histologic findings confirmed the clinical impression that this was an epidermoid carcinoma. The patient was treated with radiation therapy, but the existing edema of the larynx never subsided following therapy, and there was a persistent discomfort in this area. Mirror laryngoscopy 3 months later revealed persistent tumor; biopsy confirmed this impression. A total laryngectomy was performed. Because of the tremendous damage to the vascularity of the local tissues, there was a wound breakdown in the postoperative period and an esophageal cutaneous fistula formed. Multiple attempts were made to close this fistula with local tissue and with a variety of myocutaneous flaps. All of these failed. During this entire period, the patient was sustained on nasogastric tube feedings. Finally, using a specially designed Silastic cover, the fistula was sealed and the patient resumed normal swallowing. He then learned esophageal speech and resumed a somewhat normal life as a laryngectomee.

Because of the enormous bills incurred and because of his own anger at the primary care physician's failure to recognize this tumor earlier, the patient sought legal consultation. His medical records were subpoenaed, and the physicians involved were interviewed. The primary care physician's early notes documented presence of a sore throat and when this did not clear after a month, indicated that the patient had been referred to an ear, nose, and throat specialist. A subsequent note indicated that the patient failed to see an ENT doctor, was still complaining of a sore throat, and was again advised to seek specialty consultation. The patient denied that the physician had ever referred him to a specialist, so the records were analyzed for their validity. A handwriting specialist was unable to determine any inconsistencies in the records, but isotope dating of the ink clearly demonstrated that all of the notes suggesting the patient referral to an ENT specialist had been written 9 to 12 months after the original notes. Medical testimony at the time of trial stated that it was the standard practice to perform complete head and neck examination, including mirror laryngoscopy, on all patients who have a sore throat that does not clear after 3 to 4 weeks of medical therapy. It was also the medical opinion that the failure to diagnose this tumor for 1 year may have contributed to the treatment failure and to the patient's ultimate complications and prolonged, difficult recovery. Physician charges for this patient totaled $18,000 and the hospital charges totaled $190,000. The patient had been hospitalized for a period of 220 days, and the entire treatment and recovery spanned a period of 2 years. The court decided in favor of the plaintiff and awarded him $2 million dollars.

The original primary care physician made two serious errors. The first was that he failed to refer a patient with a chronic sore throat for a complete head and neck examination when the sore throat failed to respond in the usual fashion to his medical treatment. The second error, which constituted a serious lapse in judgment, was that he falsified his records—an inexcusable action.

Figure 6.1 is an algorithm for the evaluation of a mucosal lesion. Every mucosal lesion is unique, and so it is difficult to compose a single algorithm that solves all problems; this one does, however,

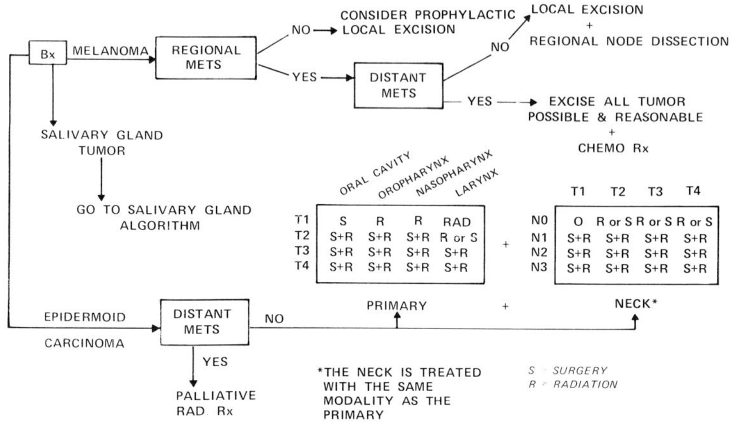

Figure 6.1. Algorithm for the evaluation of a mucosal lesion. T = tumor; N = node.

give some insight into some of the thought processes involved in identifying these complex tumors.

SALIVARY GLAND CANCER

The major salivary glands are the parotid, the submandibular, and sublingual glands. There are, in addition, thousands of single, isolated, minor salivary glands throughout the mucosal surfaces of the head and neck. Salivary gland tumors constitute about 3% of all head and neck tumors; 80% involve the parotid gland. Eighty percent of parotid tumors, 50% of submandibular and sublingual tumors, and only 20% of the minor salivary gland tumors are benign. The most common benign salivary gland tumor is a pleomorphic adenoma, often called a benign mixed tumor. The other benign tumors include the papillary cystadenoma lymphomatosum, usually called a Warthin's tumor, and the oncocytoma. Malignant tumors include mucoepidermoid carcinoma, acinous cell carcinoma, adenocarcinoma, epidermoid carcinoma, and undifferentiated carcinoma.

Most salivary gland tumors present as an asymptomatic mass. They do not cause pain and they do not noticeably interfere with salivary gland function. If a parotid tumor causes facial nerve paralysis, it is malignant. Metastatic disease in the neck is also a sign of malignancy. These tumors should not be biopsied. The patient must be evaluated, and the entire tumor excised. There are two main reasons why biopsy must be avoided. First, the facial nerve is intricately related to the parotid gland, and any incisions around the parotid gland, without first identifying the facial nerve, may risk injury to this important

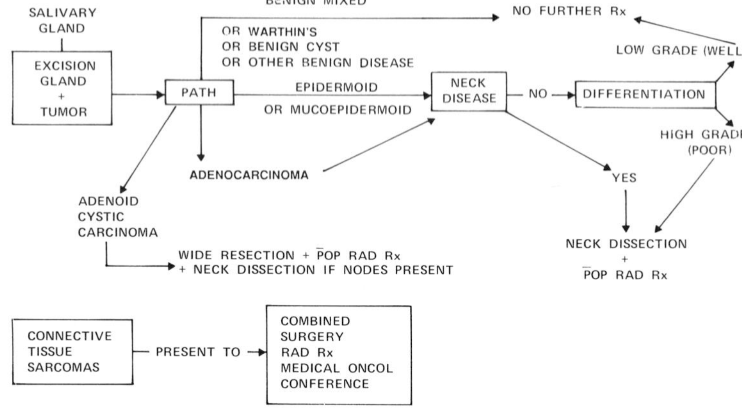

Figure 6.2. Algorithm for the evaluation of a salivary gland lesion.

structure. Second, the most common tumor is the pleomorphic adenoma. If any tumor cells spill into the local tissues, multiple adenomas will occur.

If the tumor involves the parotid gland, the facial nerve is identified and the tumor removed. If a branch of the facial nerve is involved or is cut, it should be reanastomosed or grafted using a section of another nerve. Generally, one of the nearby sensory cutaneous branches of C2, C3, or C4 is used. The greater auricular nerve is most commonly chosen. Nerve grafts work well when grafting is performed at the initial surgery; they do not work as well when performed at later dates.

Malignant salivary gland tumors are also removed with a cuff of normal tissue. Cervical metastases are treated by lymph node dissections. Patients with highly malignant tumors often receive postoperative radiation therapy.

Figure 6.2 is an algorithm for evaluating a salivary gland lesion.

THYROID CANCER

Thyroid cancer is another neoplasm occurring in the neck. Benign goiters were once very common in midwestern states, where iodinized salts were rare in nature. With the current availability of iodine-containing foods, benign goiter is uncommon in the United States. Most goiters are managed medically. However, if a goiter becomes so large that it interferes with breathing or swallowing or if it becomes cosmetically disfiguring, it can be removed surgically.

Most thyroid malignancies present as an asymptomatic mass in the thyroid gland. Benign nodules are found in approximately 3% to 5%

of the population and malignant nodules in 0.15%. In a patient with a thyroid mass, a number of factors and circumstances are suggestive of a malignancy rather than of a benign nodule. These include the following: (1) male, (2) youth, (3) positive family history of thyroid cancer, (4) history of radiation exposure, (5) enlargement of thyroid nodule, (6) single versus multiple nodules, (7) firmness of nodule, (8) fixation, (9) local adenopathy, (10) hoarseness, and (11) distant spread. Low-dose radiation to the head and neck was given to a number of patients in the late 1940s and early 1950s to reduce the size of the thymus gland. This was of no benefit to the thymus but increased the subsequent risk of developing carcinoma of the thyroid 30-fold. Therefore, anyone with a history of low-dose radiation therapy to the neck (500 to 1500 rad) must be suspected of having a thyroid malignancy and must be followed carefully with an annual examination. Certainly, a thyroid mass and a history of radiation therapy is highly suggestive of malignancy.

A number of diagnostic tools are available to evaluate thyroid nodules. Radioisotope scanning is used to evaluate a thyroid nodule's activity. Probably the best scan for evaluating the thyroid is iodine-123, but technetium-99m is also commonly used. If the nodule is found to be hyperactive (the so-called hot nodule), the probability of a malignancy is extremely low. If the nodule is cold, it must be evaluated further to rule out a neoplasm. Ultrasound will distinguish thyroid cysts from thyroid masses. The incidence of carcinoma associated with a cyst is less than that with a homogeneous noncystic lesion. Tumors can occur in association with a cyst as well.

Diagnosis

The best diagnostic procedure available today is a fine needle biopsy or aspiration. Fine needle aspiration is becoming a common technique for cytologic evaluation of the neck and thyroid masses. A No. 22 to No. 25 needle is placed on a 10- or 20-ml syringe. The needle is inserted transcutaneously into the mass. The plunger is pulled back forcefully as the needle is moved around within the mass. The needle is removed and 2 to 5 ml of saline or other physiologic solution is aspirated through the needle into the syringe. The contents of the syringe are then injected onto a glass slide or onto a piece of filter paper. The materials are processed and stained for cytologic detail. The cells are evaluated for cytologic changes. Experienced physicians, with the aid of experienced pathologists, can make a positive diagnosis in 80% to 90% of malignant cervical and thyroid tumors. If the aspiration confirms the presence of malignancy, the lesion needs to be treated as outlined later. An aspirate showing benign cytology usually excludes the presence of a malignancy. Figure 6.3 is an algorithm for the evaluation of a thyroid nodule.

The next step is to supress the thyroid using thyroxine with a dose of 100 to 150 μg of tetraiodothyronine (T_4). If the nodule decreases

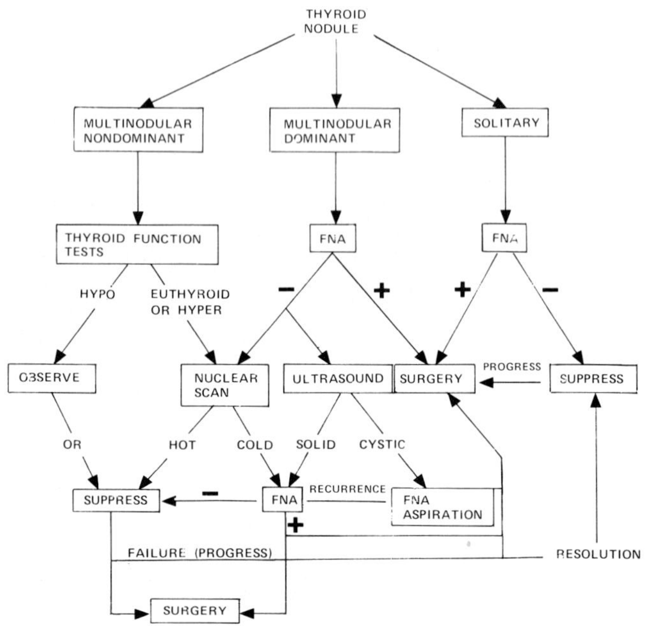

Figure 6.3. Fine needle aspiration (FNA) is an excellent diagnostic technique that has low morbidity. We use this on virtually every thyroid nodule. Figure 6.3 shows the indications for FNA in patients who present with thyroid nodules. Thyroid nodules can be classified as solitary (as shown on the right), or multinodular (as shown on the left). The solitary nodule is more likely to be malignant than the multinodular nodule; therefore, FNA is the first diagnostic step taken. If this is positive, surgery is recommended. If it is negative, the patient is put on thyroid suppression; usually, the nodule regresses or at least does not progress. If there is progression of the nodule, then surgery is recommended regardless of the FNA result. If the patient has a multinodular goiter, it is important to determine whether there is a dominant nodule present or whether all nodules are the same size. If there is not a dominant nodule, then thyroid function studies are performed. Patients who are found to be hyperthyroid should undergo a nuclear scan. A few patients may be found to have cold areas, in which case these lesions are suspicious for malignancy and FNA is indicated. Patients who have a dominant nodule as part of their multinodular goiter, should have an FNA of this nodule. If the FNA is positive, surgery is recommended. If the FNA is negative, a nuclear scan and an ultrasound are recommended. Patients who have cold areas on the nuclear scan or have solid areas on the ultrasound, require an FNA because these lesions are more likely to be malignant. If on the ultrasound the lesion is found to be cystic, the fluid should be aspirated. If there is a recurrence of the fluid, these lesions should be reaspirated.

**Table 6.1 Classification of Thyroid
Carcinomas**

Carcinoma
  Papillary adenocarcinoma
    Pure papillary
    Mixed papillary and follicular
  Follicular carcinoma
    Pure follicular
    Clear cell
    Oxyphil cell
  Medullary carcinoma
  Undifferentiated carcinoma (anaplastic)
    Small cell
    Giant cell
  Epidermoid carcinoma

Other malignant tumors
  Lymphoma
  Sarcoma
  Secondary tumor

in size or remains unchanged, it is probably a benign nodule. If it grows in size, it must be highly suspect for malignancy. Masses that are either positive on fine needle aspiration for malignancy or fail to be suppressed on thyroxine treatment require surgery. The standard operation for diagnosing a thyroid malignancy is a lobectomy. If the frozen section confirms that a malignancy is present, a thyroidectomy, preserving the contralateral parathyroid glands, is performed. Any remaining thyroid gland should be ablated with iodine-131 therapy, and the patient maintained on 100 to 150 μg of T_4 suppression for the remainder of his or her life. The combination of all three treatment modalities—that is, surgery, ^{131}I, and thyroid suppression—yields the lowest recurrence rate. If metastases are present in the neck, they should be removed.

Several factors make local, regional, and distant recurrence more likely. Patients over the age of 50 years are much more likely to have a more malignant disease. Multifocal disease and larger tumors carry a worse prognosis, as does local invasion of surrounding structures.

Table 6.1 is a useful classification of thyroid carcinomas.

Prognosis

By far the most common tumors are papillary adenocarcinomas. These carry a favorable prognosis, with 5-year control rates of 95% and 20-year survival rates of 80%. Follicular carcinomas are a little more aggressive, with a 5-year control rate of 85% and a 20-year survival rate of 50%. Medullary carcinoma is clearly more aggressive, with 5-year control rates of 50% and 20-year survival rates of 40%. An-

Table 6.2 Laboratory Findings in Common Thyroid Conditions

MEDICAL CONDITION	LABORATORY TESTS				
	T_3 (nd/dL)	T_3 Uptake (%)	T_4 (µg/dL)	Normalized Free T_4 Conc. Index Index (µg/dL)	TSH (µU/mL)
Normal	65–220	35–45	4.5–12.0	3.4–12.7	≤10
Hypothyroidism					
Subclinical	Normal	Normal	Normal	Normal	↑
Early	Normal	Normal to ↓	↓	↓	↑
Advanced	↓ (< 100)	↓	↓ (~2 µg/dL)	↓	↑ (May be >20 M/mL
Hyperthyroidism	(Avg. of 700–800)		(Avg. of ~20 µg/dL)		
Graves' disease	↑ (Usually to a greater extent than T_4) greater	↑	↑	↑	↓
Toxic multinodular goiter	High normal to ↑	High normal to ↑	High normal to ↑	High normal to ↑	Normal to ↓
Hyperfunctioning adenoma	↑ (Often causes T_3 toxicosis)	↑	↑	↑	↓
Secondary	↑	↑	↑	↑	↑
Thyroiditis					
Subacute	↑ Early ↓ Later	↑ Early ↓ Later	↑ Early ↓ Later	↑ Early ↓ Later	↓ Early ↑ Later

Chronic	All indexes for 2–5 mo (except TSH which is ↓), often followed by a self-limited phase of hypothyroidism. This pattern may repeat itself again and again.				
Early Hashimoto's	Normal	Normal first ↓ Later	Normal first ↓ Later	Normal first ↓ Later	↑
Later Hashimoto's	Normal first ↓ Later	↓	↓	↓	↑
Supplementation					
Thyroid extract USP 120–180 mg	Normal	Normal	Normal	Normal	Normal to ↓
Levothyroxine 150 μg	↓	Normal	Normal to slight ↑	Normal	Normal to ↓
Liothyronine 50 μg	↑	↓	↓	↓	Normal to ↓
Liotrix (T$_4$/T$_3$ = 4/1)2 U	Normal to	Normal	Normal	Normal	Normal to ↓
Suppression	As above; object is to ↓ TSH. If adequately suppressed, radioactive iodine uptake by the thyroid gland should be <5% of the control value.				
Cancer	All indexes are normal unless it is a rare functional tumor or much of the normal tissue has been destroyed by compression, or if inflammation results in thyroiditis.				

TSH = thyroid stimulating hormone

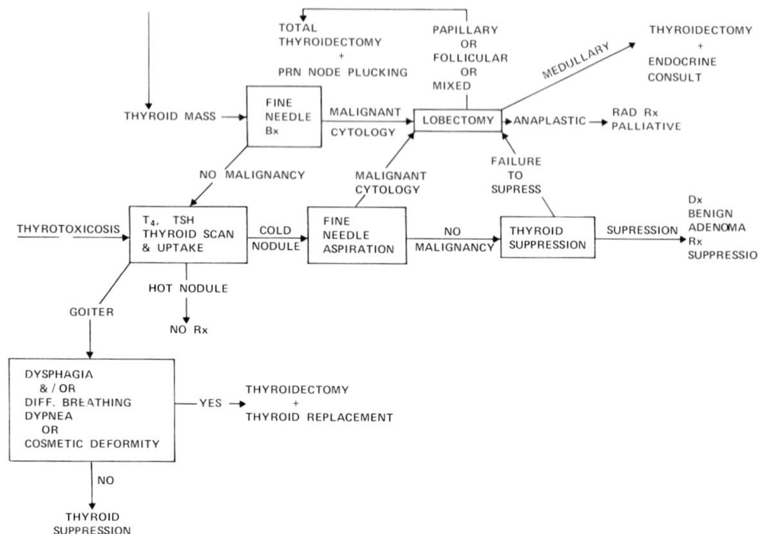

Figure 6.4. Algorithm for evaluation and treatment of a thyroid mass. Bx = biopsy; Rx = radiotherapy; Dx = diagnosis.

aplastic carcinoma is so aggressive that it is uncommon for a patient to live more than 1 year. In fact, it is so aggressive that many surgeons will not perform a thyroidectomy once this diagnosis has been made. External beam radiation therapy and chemotherapy are used only for aggressive, out-of-control tumors.

Figure 6.4 is an algorithm for the evaluation of a thyroid lesion and Table 6.2 is a chart of laboratory findings in several medical conditions.

SKIN CANCER

Skin cancer is a major medical problem in light-complected patients who have had significant UV (sun) light exposure. The two most common malignancies are basal cell cancer and epidermoid or squamous cell cancer. Melanoma is also related to sun exposure but occurs much less commonly.

Basal Cell and Epidermoid Cancer

Basal cell and epidermoid cancers occur primarily on the sun-exposed surfaces of the skin; 90% occur on the head and neck. Patients recognize skin cancer as a raised tumor or a nonhealing sore. Dermatologists are the most skilled diagnosticians for skin cancer, particularly in its early phases. Most tumors can be recognized early and treated with cryotherapy (liquid nitrogen), 5-flurouracil, or curettage and electrodesiccation. More advanced, more aggressive, or recurrent tumors are best treated surgically. Although clinical diagnosis can be extremely accurate, a biopsy is generally made to confirm the tumor type and to discover something about its biologic behavior. Most tumors have a well-defined border. They can be safely excised with a 2-mm margin of normal tissue. The defect is closed with a skin graft or a local skin flap.

Certain tumors are known to be more invasive. These include recurrent basal cell tumors, sclerosing or fibrosing basal cell tumors, and large or invasive epidermoid tumors. These tumors must be removed with microscopic-controlled margins, a technique known as

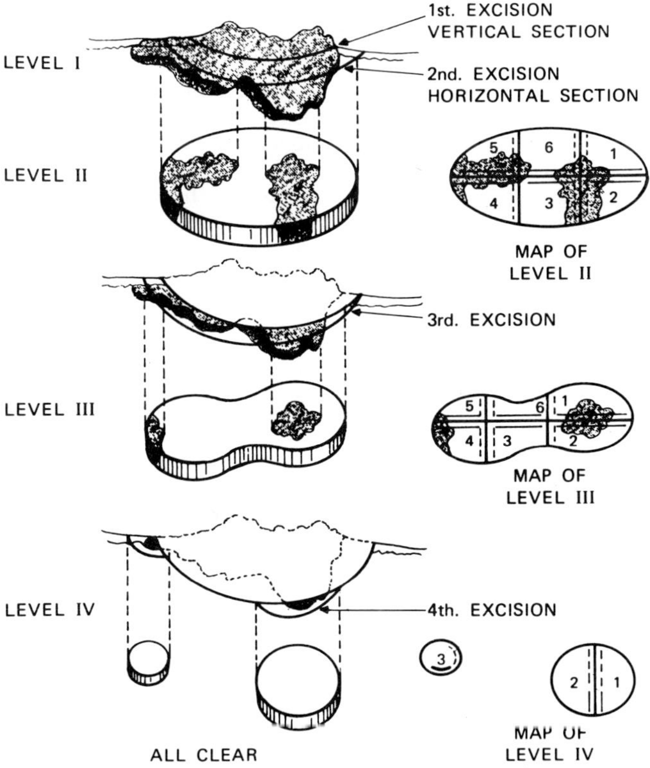

Figure 6.5. Mohs' chemosurgery. The drawings on the left depict a cutaneous tumor at successive levels of excision. The drawings on the right are the maps maintaining orientation for the frozen section examination.

Mohs' chemosurgery. Although chemosurgery is a misnomer as the technique is applied today, it does distinguish the manner in which the frozen sections are done. The technique of Mohs' chemosurgery (Fig. 6.5) is so important to successful skin cancer surgery that it is worth describing. The clinically evident tumor is removed. Next, a thin slice of tissue from the remaining skin bed is excised. This is cut into pieces approximately 1 × 1 cm. A careful map is drawn to maintain orientation. Each of the sectioned pieces is laid flat and frozen, after which a thin section is cut. This is placed on a microscope slide, stained, and examined. If tumor is found, the respective area is identified on the map. Additional excisions are made and treated identically. This process is continued until no additional tumor is identified. The technique is time-consuming and is indicated only for tumors for which local control is difficult. This technique gives the surgeon the maximum chance of removing all the tumor while removing the minimum amount of normal healthy tissue.

Primary basal cell cancers have a surgical cure rate of at least 95%. The surgical cure rate for recurrent or sclerosing basal cell cancer is only 50%. Using the frozen section control as developed by Mohs, the 50% cure rate has been raised to at least 98%.

Occasionally, a patient will allow a skin tumor to grow for years until it involves a major portion of the face. In this situation, wide surgical excision with the same microscopically controlled frozen sections is performed. The defects are closed with skin grafts or large

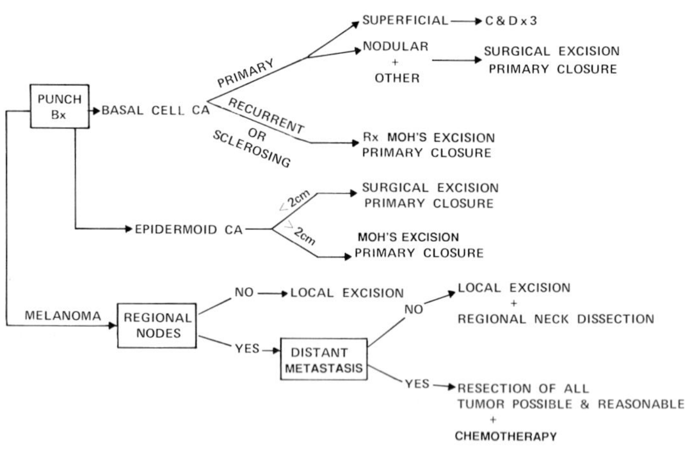

Figure 6.6.   Algorithm for the evaluation of a skin lesion. C + D = curettage and dissection; Bx = biopsy.

local skin flaps. Defects involving the loss of an ear, an eye, or the nose are reconstructed with prostheses.

Metastatic basal cell cancer is extremely rare. Advanced epidermoid cancers on the skin will, however, metastasize. Lymph node dissection and radiation are then necessary.

Figure 6.6 is an algorithm for the evaluation of a skin lesion.

Melanoma

Melanoma is a deadly tumor that affects both males and females, young and old. It can be rapidly fatal. It may arise in a previously pigmented skin lesion or may arise de novo. It also occurs on mucosal surfaces and on the retina. Often an inflammatory response is present around it. Diagnosis is made by excisional biopsy; a punch biopsy or an incisional biopsy is less desirable. Histologic examination of the entire primary cutaneous lesion is important for diagnosis, treatment, and prognosis. Very superficial lesions of melanoma metastasize infrequently. Initially, invasion was described by the histologic depth of invasion. Clark characterized the depth of invasion as levels I through V, with level I being a superficial tumor and level V a deeply invasive tumor. Unfortunately, pathologists examining the same slides would interpret these levels differently, creating difficulties with inconsistency. Breslow categorized invasion simply by measuring the depth of the skin invasion. A melanoma that has invaded 0 to 0.75 mm is unlikely to metastasize, one that has invaded 0.75 to 1.5 mm is likely to metastasize, and one that has invaded deeper than 1.5 mm is very likely to metastasize. This system seems to be easier to use and gives a more consistent interpretation. Hematogenous metastasis is common with deeply invasive lesions. A thorough laboratory and radioisotope examination should be performed on all patients.

The primary tumor is treated by surgery. Wide local incision is needed, with margins of 1 to 3 cm being required for superficial tumors. Advanced tumors require optimal margins of up to 5 cm, although this is often not possible on the head and neck. If regional lymph nodes are involved, they should be removed. Prophylactic removal of the lymph notes is controversial; it does not affect the ultimate cure rate, but it is a very important prognosticator. The surgeon and the patient must themselves decide if the added information justifies the additional surgery. Postoperative radiation therapy, chemotherapy, and immunotherapy are often used.

There are now many radiographic techniques to examine the head and neck. Plain films, CT scanning, and MRI are the three most important modalities. Each has its own value and place in evaluating head and neck disease. Table 6.3 was constructed by Robert Tien, MD, a neuroradiologist at University of California, San Diego, and compares the value of these three modalities for the most common head and neck radiographic requests.

Table 6.3 Comparison of Radiographic Modalities for Common Head and Neck Evaluations

	PLAIN FILM	CT	MRI
Cerebellopontine angle	No use	Little benefit	Very useful
Skull base	No use	Very useful	Very useful
Temporal bone	Little benefit	Very useful	Useful
Nasopharynx	No use	Useful	Very useful
Maxillary sinus	Some	Very useful	Useful
Paranasal sinuses	Some	Very useful	Useful
Facial fracture	Useful	Very useful	Little benefit
Mandibular fracture	Very useful	Useful	No use
Laryngeal fracture	No use	Very useful	No use
Laryngeal tumor	Contrast laryngogram useful	Useful	Very useful
Cervical nodes	No use	Very useful	Very useful
Thyroid neoplasm	No use	*Useful	*Useful

*Ultrasound is useful too.

CHAPTER 7

Facial Plastic and Reconstructive Surgery

Facial plastic and reconstructive surgery of the head and neck is a broad and fascinating field. Two major topics will be covered in this chapter: maxillofacial trauma and cosmetic surgery. With regard to the first topic, the emergency department—the place where the resident is most likely to encounter trauma—can be a terrifying place at times, filled as it is with the startling and often tragic effects of human violence and with the need to make important decisions accurately and immediately.

MAXILLOFACIAL TRAUMA

Facial trauma is very common in today's society. This undoubtedly reflects the fact that many individuals drive under the influence of alcohol or other intoxicating agents, and that others have suffered various forms of personal violence.

Evaluation (Fig. 7.1) is the key to the diagnosis and treatment of facial trauma. A soft tissue injury requires thorough evaluation. Before examining the patient, the attending physician must become familiar with the underlying muscles, nerves (especially the peripheral motor branches of the facial nerve), major vessels, course of the salivary ducts, and anatomy of the underlying mucosa along with the underlying bony skeleton.

Physical Examination

The skin must be examined for lacerations, abrasions, and contusions. Determination is made if the wound is clean or dirty. Whenever an open wound is present, the patient must be adequately immunized against tetanus. Underlying tissues must be examined. Bleeding vessels are controlled with cautery, suture, or pressure. Lacerated muscles will alter facial movement and must be reapproximated with 4-0 Vicryl or Dexon sutures. Injury to sensory nerves should be noted, but no

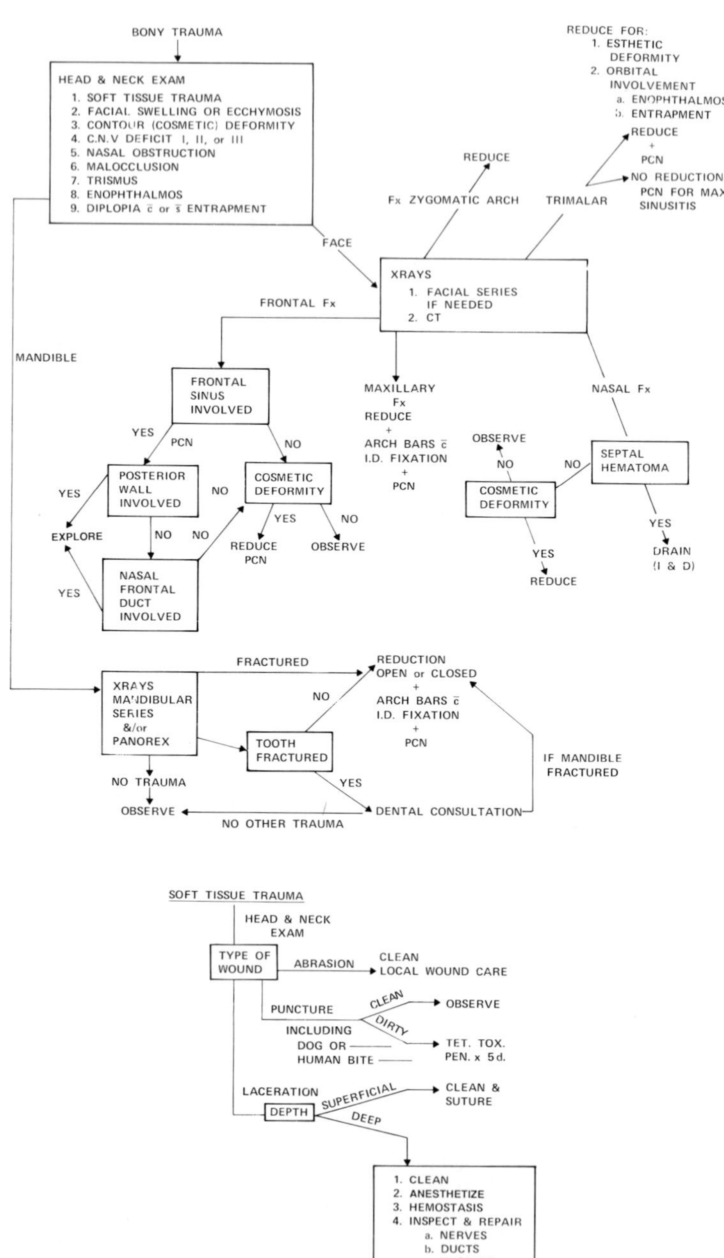

Figure 7.1. Algorithm for evaluation of facial trauma.

166

therapy is needed; the patient recovers from most sensory nerve losses spontaneously. Injury to motor nerves must be diagnosed and repaired. Normally, the cut nerve ends are identified and sutured together under the microscope with 8-0 or 10-0 monofilament nylon sutures. If a salivary duct is cut, the ends should be found, the duct cannulated with Silastic tubing, and the ends sutured together over the Silastic cannula.

X-Ray Examination

The cervical and facial bones can be evaluated by inspection, palpation, conventional X-ray examination, and CT scanning. In the 1970s, the only radiographic examinations available were conventional X rays. Physicians trained prior to and during that period became very skilled at making diagnoses based on standard X-ray views, occasionally in conjunction with tomography. With the advent of CT scanning, the practice in many institutions has changed. For many situations, such as head trauma, some facial trauma, and laryngotracheal trauma, the CT scan is believed to be superior to X-ray views. It is my opinion that for most simple facial fractures, such as a mandibular fracture, the conventional X-ray examination is superior because it is less expensive, easier to perform, and subjects the patient to less radiation. On the other hand, if the injury is complex or involves areas such as the brain, the orbit, or the larynx—sites where conventional X rays are difficult to interpret—then the CT scan is superior. Because of the variability in equipment and physician expertise, different institutions and individual physicians will rely on the different radiographic modalities according to varying circumstances.

If there is any possibility of cervical spine injury, a cross-table lateral X-ray examination is made first. If no fractures are seen, a cervical spinal series is obtained. Suspected skull trauma is evaluated by a skull series.

For facial fractures, a facial series is ordered with the patient in the upright position. This should include five views: posteroanterior (PA), Caldwell, Waters, submental vertical (SMV), and lateral X rays. Figure 7.2 shows the orientation for four of the five facial series of X rays and indicates normal bony anatomy. Figure 7.3 is a normal facial series showing all five X-ray views. Correlate these X rays with a skull or with Figure 7.2. Tomographic studies and CT scans are ordered only if additional detail is needed. The mandible can be evaluated by inspection and with several different X-ray views. The teeth and the patient's dental occlusion are examined. If there is any suspicion of a fracture, an X-ray study is done. The easiest is a Panorex, which is generally performed by the dental service. A normal Panorex is shown in Figure 7.4. Conventional mandibular X-ray views include a posteroanterior and right and left oblique views. A special view of the mandibular condyle is sometimes included. The Caldwell view on the facial series also shows the condyle well. Normal

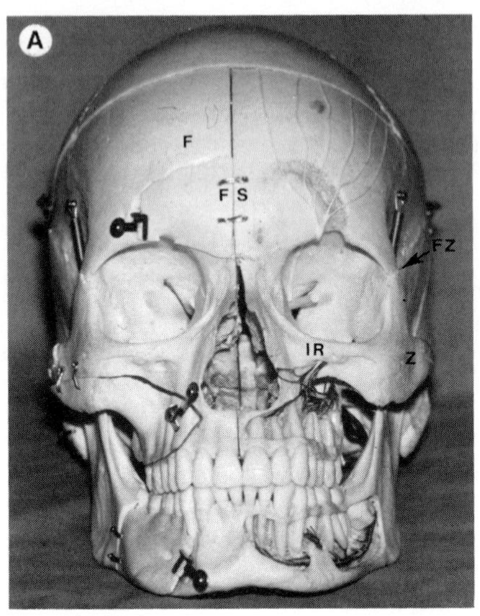

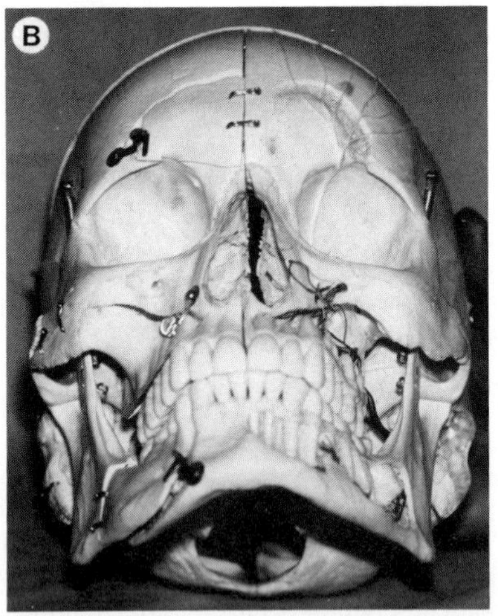

Figure 7.2.   Facial fractures. These four photographs show a skeleton as it would be positioned for a facial X-ray series. (A) Posteroanterior view. (B) Waters view. *(Continued on p. 169.)*

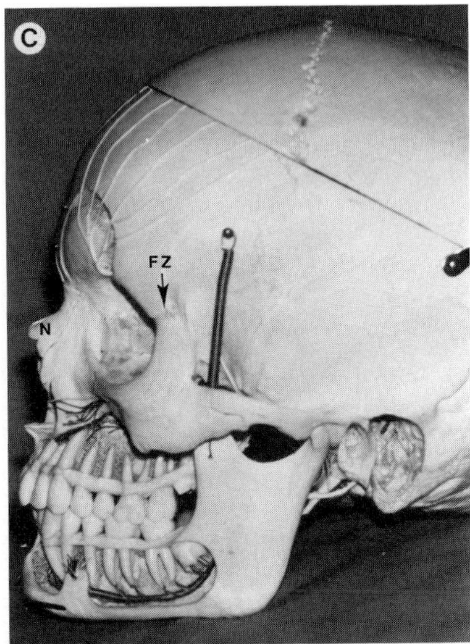

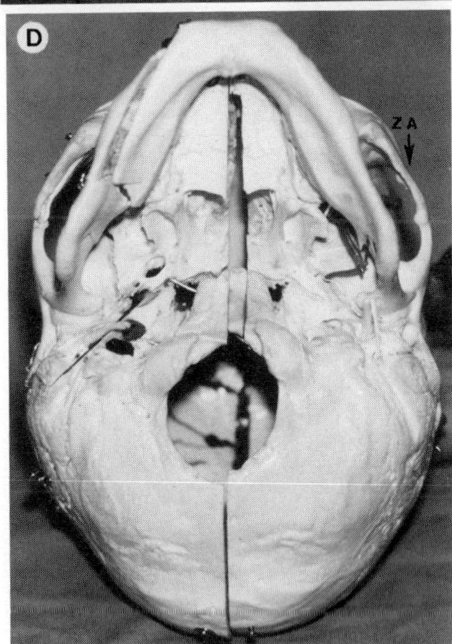

Figure 7.2. **(continued)** (C) Lateral view. (D) Submental vertical view. (F = frontal bone, FS = frontal sinus, FZ = frontozygomatic suture, Z = zygoma, IR = infraorbital rim, N = nasal bones, ZA = zygomatic arch.)

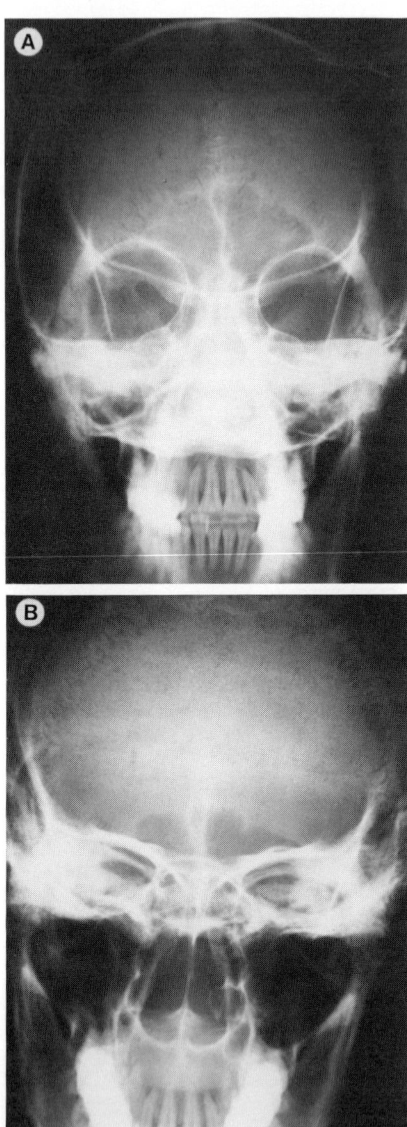

Figure 7.3.   Facial fracture X rays. These X rays are taken with the patient sitting upright and are best performed with equipment especially designed for head and neck X rays. (A) Posteroanterior view. (B) Caldwell view. *(Continued on p. 171.)*

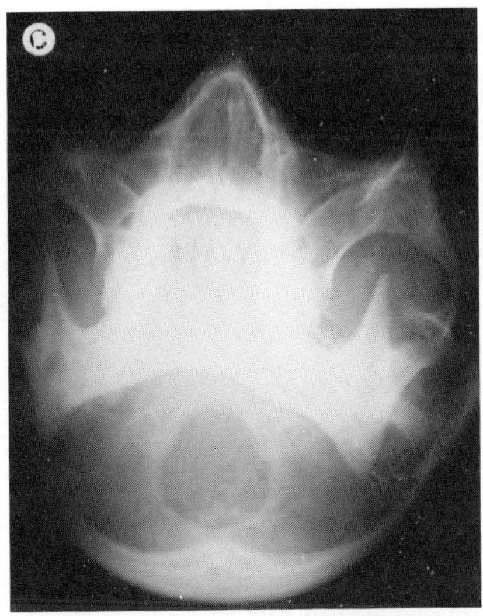

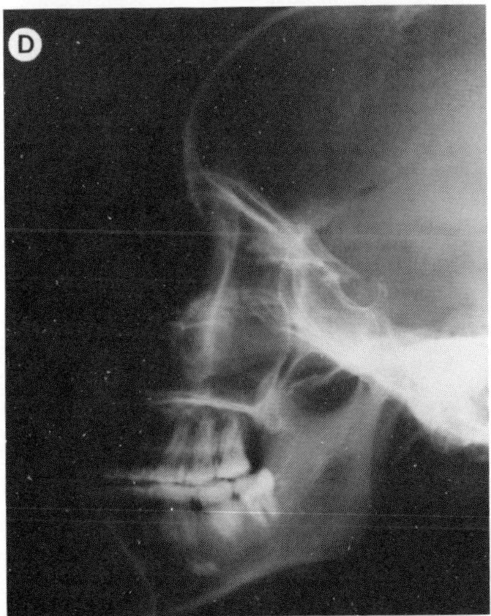

Figure 7.3. **(continued)** (C) Waters' view. (D) Lateral view. *(Continued on p. 172.)*

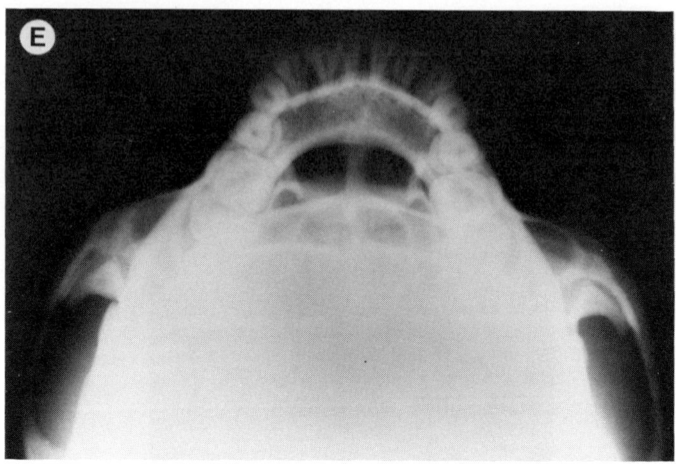

Figure 7.3. (continued) (E) Submental vertical view. Identify all the structures labeled in Figure 7.2.

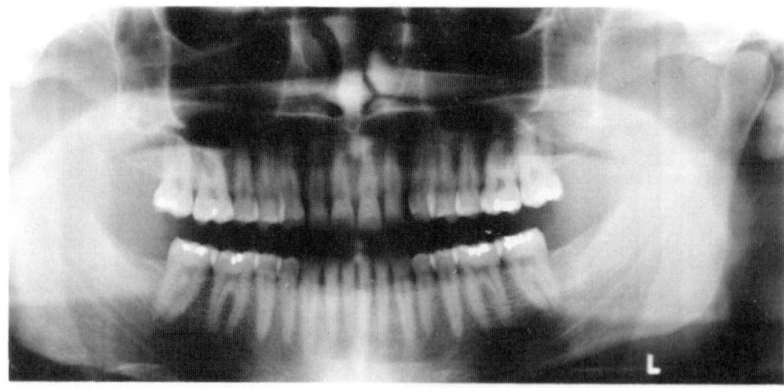

Figure 7.4. Panorex of a normal mandible with good, healthy dentition. The left mandibular condyle can be seen very well. The angle and the body of the mandible and maxillary sinuses are also well seen, but the symphysis is slightly fuzzy.

mandibular X rays are shown in Figure 7.5. Nasal X rays have not been useful because false-positive and false-negative results have been too common. Figure 7.6 is a good example of the ambiguous results frequently obtained with nasal X rays.

The decision to reduce a nasal fracture is entirely a clinical decision and is not affected by X-ray findings. X rays should not be ordered to evaluate a nasal fracture; they will not affect a clinical decision to reduce or not reduce the fracture. The only reason to obtain nasal X rays is for medico–legal purposes, which is not a sufficient reason.

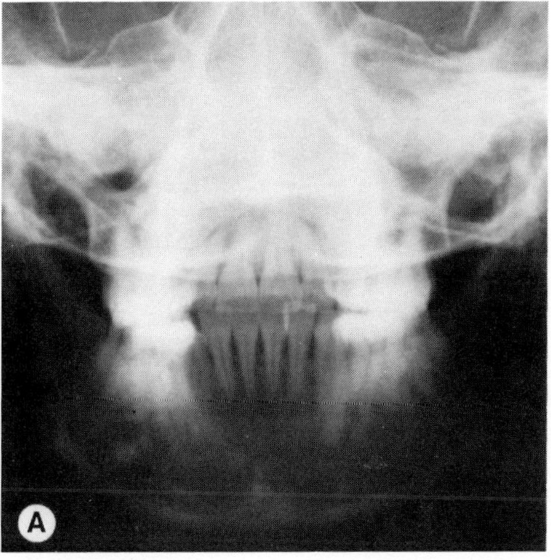

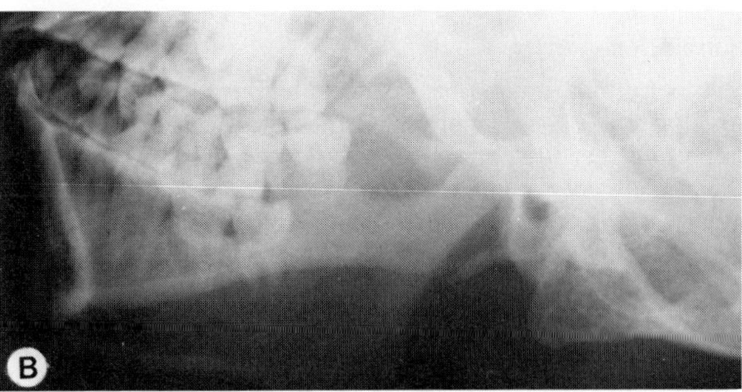

Figure 7.5. Mandibular X rays are more easily obtained than Panorex films unless the hospital has a dental service. The standard views are shown here. (A) Posteroanterior view. (B) Left oblique view.

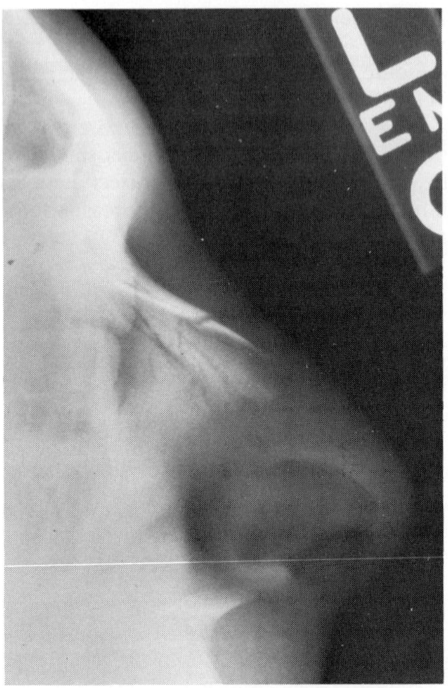

Figure 7.6. Nasal X ray of patient who was hit on the nose. The X ray is very clear, but is there a nasal fracture? Clinically there was not. Nasal X rays are not helpful evaluating nasal trauma.

Eye Examination

Ocular and periorbital trauma necessitates that vision be checked. It is far superior to use the proper charts for testing vision rather than simply reporting that the patient can read a newspaper without difficulty. Each eye is checked independently and extraocular movements and pupillary constriction evaluated. The patient is questioned about double vision (diplopia). Look for enophthalmus and examine the retina. Do not dilate the pupil for retinoscopy, as this can adversely affect the evaluation of head trauma.

Ear Examination

Hearing is tested grossly with tuning forks; examine the external auditory canal for lacerations and blood. The tympanic membranes should be checked for lacerations and a hemotympanum, and the nose examined for bleeding or a cerebrospinal fluid leak.

Treatment of Maxillofacial Injuries

Consultation with a head and neck surgeon is strongly recommended if there are any questions. The principles of treatment are as follows. Soft tissue wounds must be cleaned. Soaps, peroxides, and alcohols damage tissue. Clean the wound with tincture of povidone-iodine and a lot of warm water. Pulsatile, copious irrigation is highly affective. Eye protection is necessary because an ever-increasing number of trauma patients are HIV or HVB positive. All dirt must be removed. If dirt has been ground into the skin, the area is anesthetized with 1% lidocaine with 1:100,000 epinephrine and the dirt removed with a scrub brush. Failure to do so completely will result in permanent tattooing. Devitalized, dead tissue should be excised. This is called debridement. The bleeding is stopped with chromic or silk ligatures or with electrocautery. Cut nerves are repaired with microscopic techniques, using 8-0 or 10-0 monofilament nylon sutures. Cut muscles are reapproximated with 4-0 Vicryl or Dexon sutures. Subcutaneous tissues are closed with 4-0 Vicryl or Dexon sutures and the skin is closed with 5-0 or 6-0 nylon or Prolene sutures.

Nasal Fractures

Bony fractures are repaired if functional or cosmetic defects exist. Nasal fractures are caused by trauma either from directly in front or, more commonly, from the side. Normally, the nose will bleed for a short period and will be tender to palpation. If the nose is crooked, the fracture should be reduced. This can be performed under local anesthesia immediately or within 7 to 10 days, when swelling is decreased. The nasal septum must be examined to rule out a septal hematoma. If a hematoma exists, it must be incised and drained within 4 to 6 hours.

Case Study: Infraorbital Rim Fracture

Figure 7.7 shows a young man who was mugged. He was brought to the emergency department. He had not lost consciousness. He could not see out of his right eye. He had no significant past medical history. On examination, there was an easily palpated right infraorbital rim fracture. Total anesthesia was present over the distribution of the infraorbital branch of the fifth cranial nerve. The eye appeared normal. Extraocular movements were normal and vision was 20/20 in both eyes. The patient could not elevate the right upper eyelid because of the swelling. A facial X-ray series was ordered (Fig. 7.8). (Evaluation of these X rays should be done before reading on.)

The infraorbital rim fracture is best seen on the Waters view. The separation of the frontozygomatic suture is poorly seen. The depressed zygomatic arch is seen clearly on the SMV view.

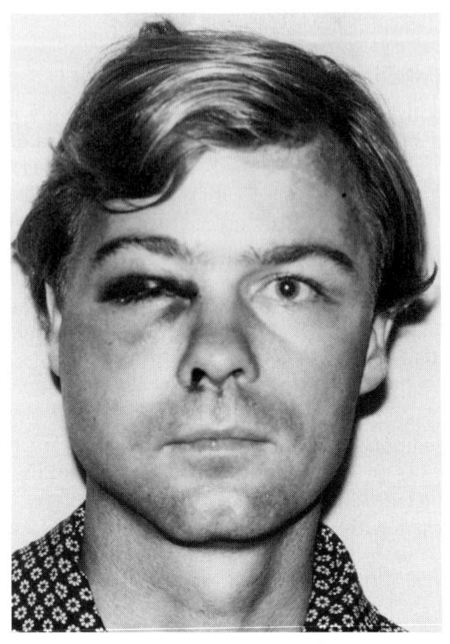

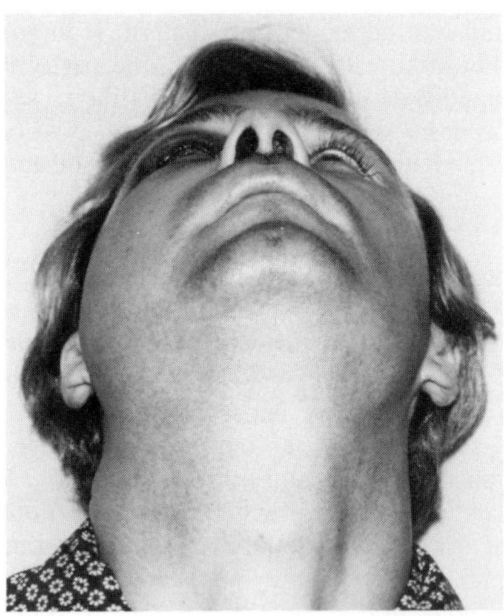

Figure 7.7. The patient's face looks relatively symmetrical, but the right side is grossly swollen. By palpation the entire malar bone was found to be depressed and a step-off infraorbital rim fracture was present.

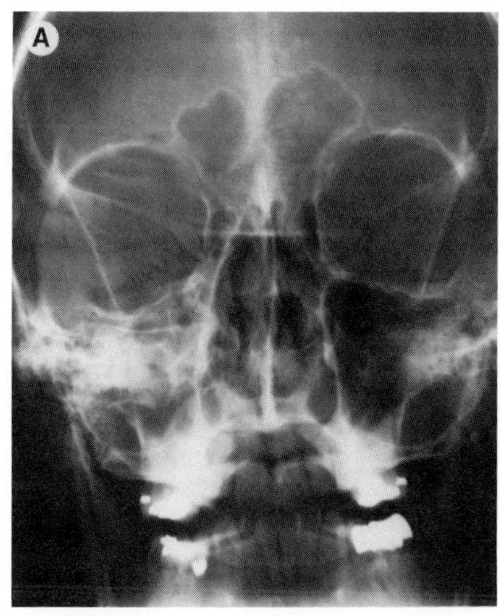

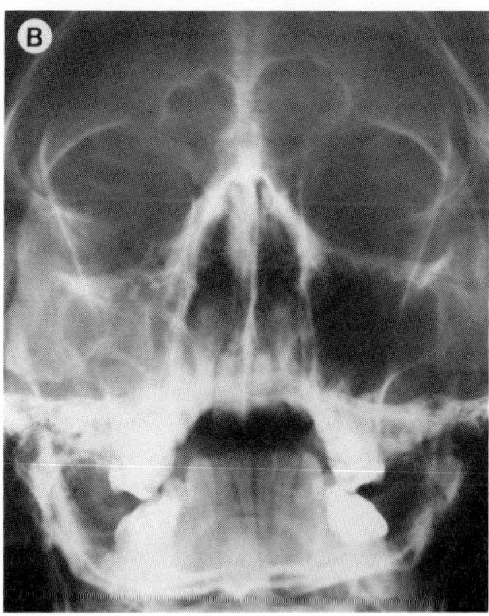

Figure 7.8. Facial X rays. (A) Posteroanterior view. (B) Waters' view. *(Continued on p. 178.)*

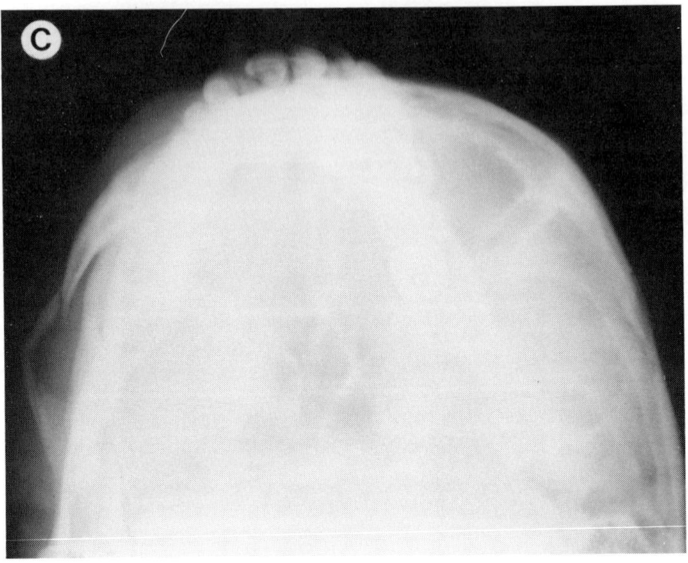

Figure 7.8. (continued) (C) SMV view. The Caldwell view is omitted here. X-ray findings include (1) large infraorbital rim step-off fracture, (2) separation of the frontozygomatic suture, (3) depressed zygomatic arch fracture, and (4) opacified right maxillary sinus fracture. Impression was of a depressed right malar fracture.

The opacified sinus seen on the Waters view is filled with blood and is supportive evidence of a maxillary fracture.

The patient was admitted to the hospital, and the next morning under general anesthesia the malar fracture was reduced and the bony fracture wired in place. Figure 7.9 shows the postreduction films. The patient recovered uneventfully. The only sequelae were two almost invisible scars from the open reductions and a dime-sized residual of anesthesia on this right cheek.

Zygomatic or Malar Fractures
Zygomatic or malar fractures are caused by a direct blow to the zygomatic arch or to the malar bone. The words malar bone and zygoma are used interchangeably. A fracture to this area can be called a malar fracture or zygomatic fracture. As with nasal fractures, some

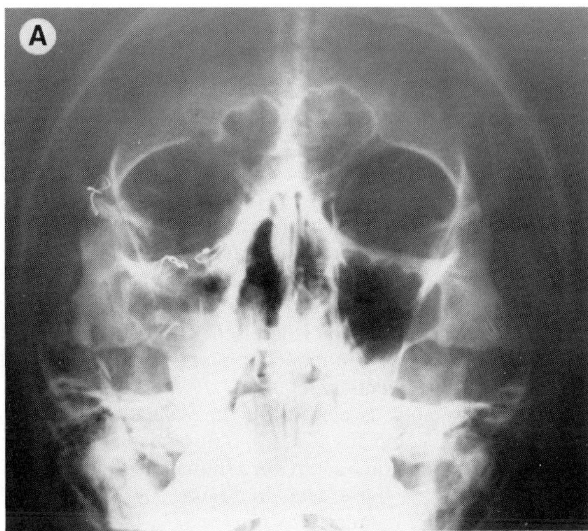

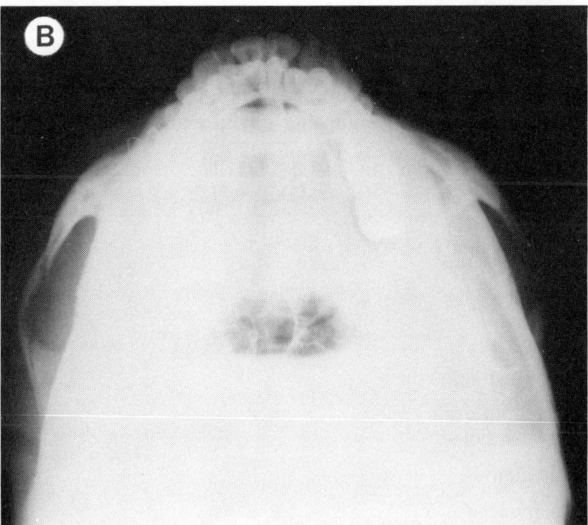

Figure 7.9. Postreduction films. (A) Waters' view. (B) SMV view. Note the wires across the frontozygomatic suture and along the infraorbital rim. There is excellent reduction of all the fractures. An air–fluid level is now present in the right maxillary sinus.

form of physical altercation is the most common cause of zygomatic fractures.

Two types of fractures are common in the zygomatic region. A direct blow to the zygomatic arch will fracture the arch alone. This is repaired by a closed reduction. A cosmetic defect or trismus may be produced by trapping of the temporalis muscle under the zygomatic arch. A blow more anteriorly to the malar eminence will cause three fractures to occur simultaneously: a fracture to the zygomatic arch, separation of the frontozygomatic suture, and an infraorbital rim fracture. The infraorbital rim fracture inevitably involves the infraorbital nerve canal. There will be a concomitant fracture of the maxillary sinus and often of the orbital floor as well. If more than 2 or 3 mm of displacement exists, reduction is advised. Often a closed reduction is possible; otherwise, an open reduction and direct wiring or plating of all the fractured fragments is required.

Computed tomography is also useful in evaluating certain facial fractures. Table 7.1 compares CT scanning and plain X-ray films. Two examples of zygomatic fractures are shown in Figure 7.10. These fractures are similar to those seen in Figure 7.8 and it might be educational to compare them.

Table 7.1 Comparison of Computed Tomography and Plain X-Ray Films in Diagnosing Facial Fractures

FACIAL FRACTURES	COMPUTED TOMOGRAPHY	PLAIN X-RAY FILMS
Anterior and posterior wall of maxillary sinus	+ +	±
Posterior displacement of maxilla zygoma	+ +	−
Anterior and posterior wall of frontal sinus	+ +	±
Zygomatic arch	+ +	+ +
Lamina papyracea	+ +	±
Lateral wall of orbit	+ +	−
Fluid, air, bone in wrong places	+ +	±

Key: + + = excellent, + = good, − = poor, and ± = sometimes good, sometimes bad.

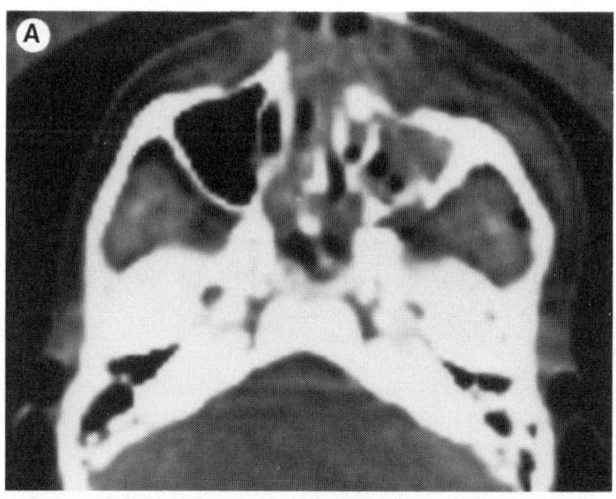

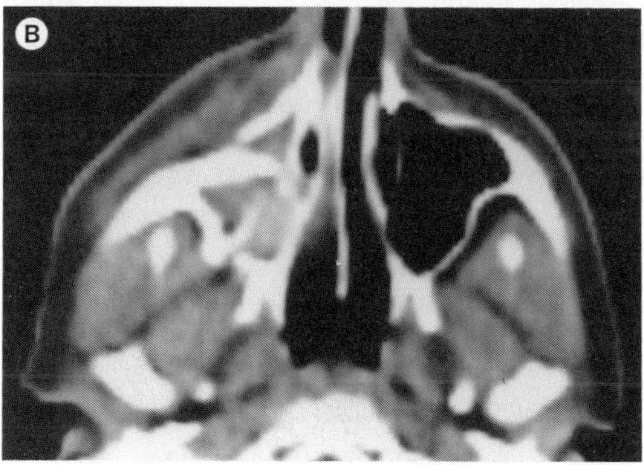

Figure 7.10. Computed tomography (CT) scans of facial fractures. (A) CT scan from a patient involved in an automobile accident. The left maxillary sinus is fractured anteriorly, posteriorly, and medially into the nose. The sinus is filled with blood. (B) CT scan from a patient involved in a dune buggy accident. The right zygoma is fractured into the maxillary sinus. There are also fractures of the anterior and posterior sinus wells. The sinus is filled with blood.

Orbital Floor Fractures

Orbital floor fractures occur with most malar fractures or from a direct blow to the eye. These fractures should be explored and repaired only if the patient has diplopia with muscle entrapment or enophthalmus. Diplopia can be caused by hematoma, by nerve injury, or by trapping one of the ocular muscles in a bony fracture. Ocular muscle entrapment can be tested by gently grasping the insertion of the involved muscle, most commonly the inferior rectus muscle, and pulling gently. If the muscle is trapped, it will not budge. If it is not entrapped, the muscle and eye will move freely. If the muscle is entrapped, the fracture should be surgically explored and the trapped muscle released from the fracture. Diplopia resulting from other causes is not improved by surgery. Enophthalmus is caused by prolapse of periorbital fat and of the eye into the maxillary sinus. These deficiencies should be repaired immediately.

Maxillary Fractures

Maxillary bone fractures are generally described as LeFort fractures I, II, or III in honor of a French physician who classified patterns of maxillary fractures. All maxillary fractures require repair because they will result in cosmetic deformity and malocclusion. Figure 7.11 shows the three classic LeFort fractures marked on a skeleton. Arch bars have been applied to the maxillary and mandibular teeth. The fractured bones are wired or plated to stable bones above the fracture. Occlusion is maintained by wiring the upper and lower teeth together. This is done by wiring metal braces, or arch bars, to the upper and lower teeth and then joining the braces together with rubber bands. This is called interdental fixation. When the maxilla or the mandible is fractured, it is crucial that the fracture heal with the teeth in optimum occlusion. Failure to do this disrupts mastication and the longevity of the teeth and, frequently, will cause temporomandibular joint dysfunction.

Mandibular Fractures

Mandibular fractures are common facial fractures. They are seen most frequently in males between the ages of 15 and 40 years. Most are caused in physical altercations. Figure 7.12 shows the nomenclature commonly used to describe fractures at various sites. The frequency of the different fractures is also shown. Mandibular X-ray examination is illustrated in Figures 7-4 and 7-5. The most important consideration in the repair of mandibular fractures is the restoration of normal dental occlusion. As with maxillary fractures, this is done by wiring braces, called arch bars, to the mandibular and maxillary teeth and then joining the bars with rubber bands. Normal occlusion is illustrated on a model in Figure 7.13A. In Figure 7.13B, arch bars have been wired to the teeth and then joined with rubberbands. Nondisplaced mandibular fractures and those involving the condyle are treated with arch bars and interdental fixation. Displaced fractures require open reduction, direct wiring or plating of the fractures, and application of arch bars with interdental fixation.

The approach to the repair of bony fractures has evolved during the past decades. The early goals of fracture repair were stabilization, generally with external casting. When this failed to achieve alignment, traction was applied and then held. As surgical repair increased in safety, open reductions with stainless steel wire fixation became popular. This still required immobilization until bony union became sufficiently strong for the bone to return to function. More recently, stronger fixation techniques have evolved. For the head and neck this involves stainless steel or titanium plates that are secured to the bone

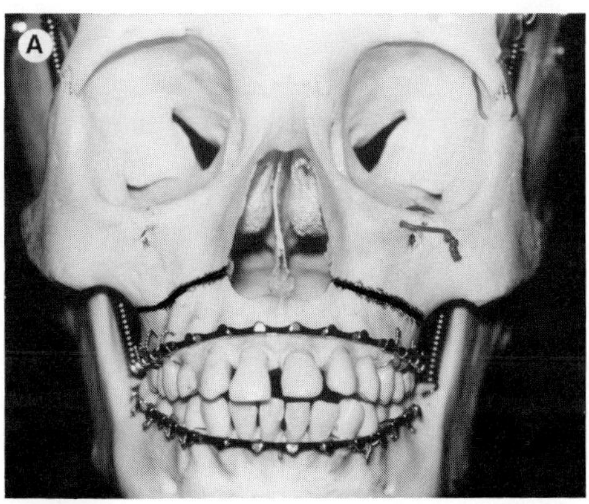

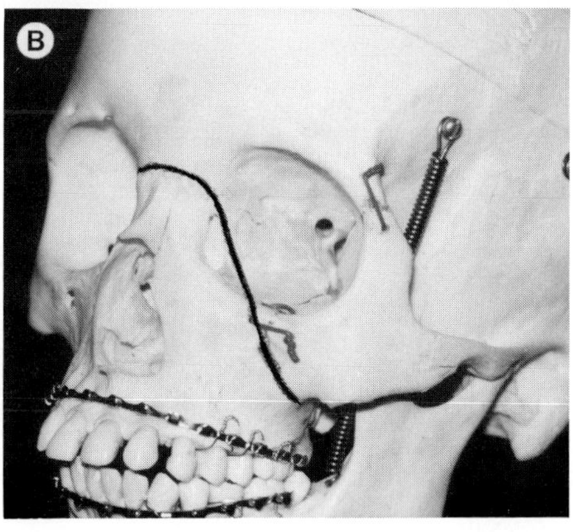

Figure 7.11. Fractures of the maxilla are frequently classified as LeFort fractures. These three photographs show the "classic" LeFort fractures. Each fracture is marked by a black line. Arch bars have been applied to the teeth. Wires have been placed showing the open reduction and internal fixation used for trimalar fractures. (A) LeFort I fracture. (B) LeFort II fracture. *(Continued on p. 183.)*

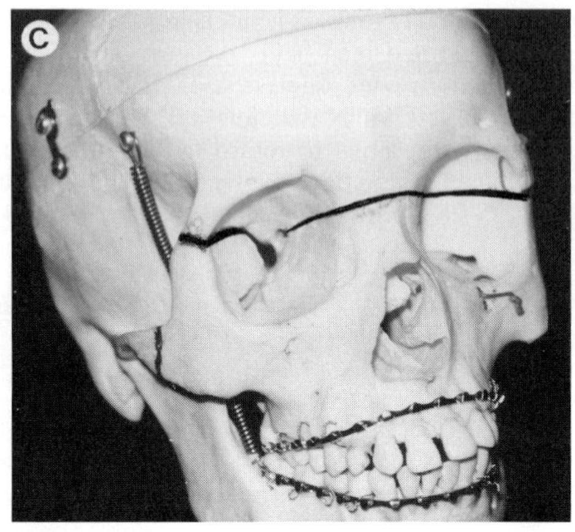

Figure 7.11. (continued) (C) LeFort III fracture.

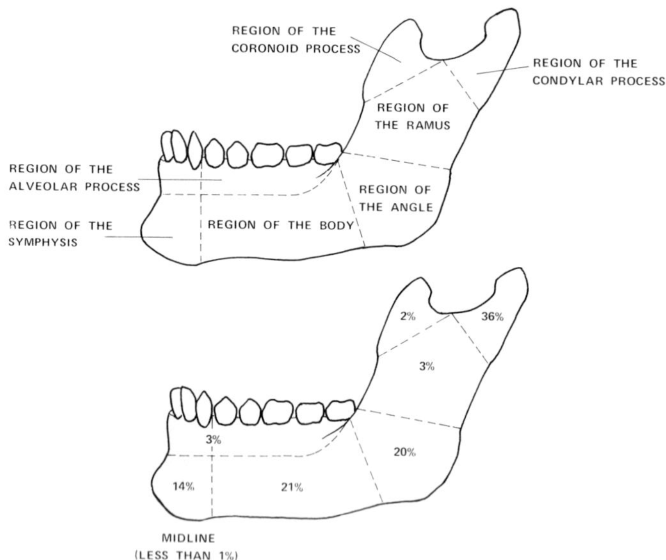

Figure 7.12.   The sites of mandibular fractures and the frequency of these fractures, from the head and neck experience at the University and VA Hospitals in San Diego.

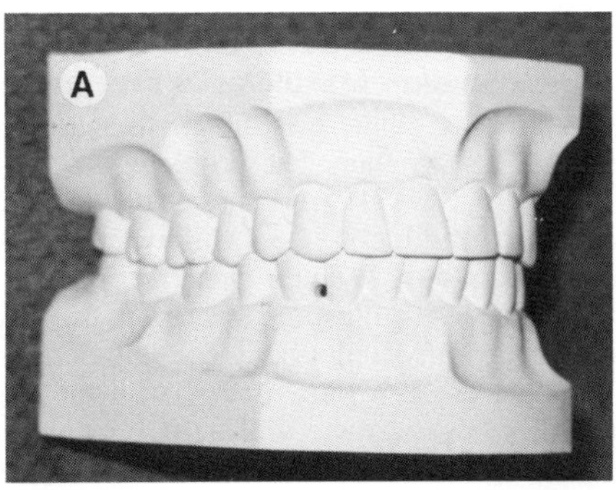

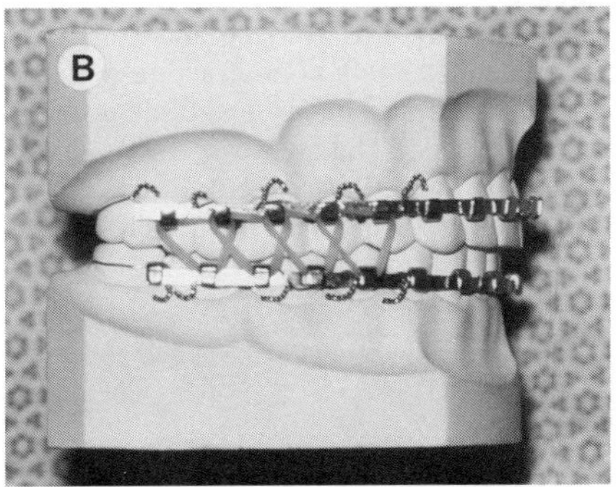

Figure 7.13. Arch bars. (A) A plaster cast model showing normal dental occlusion. Occlusion primarily involves the molar teeth, that is, the grinding surfaces of the teeth. (B) Arch bars are applied and interdental fixation is obtained with rubber bands.

with screws. This repair technique is so strong that immobilization requirements have been reduced.

In facial trauma, this has changed the approach to mandibular and maxillary fractures. Past techniques required 3 to 6 weeks of interdental fixation to insure healing with proper dental occlusion. With the advent of plates, many fractures do not require any interdental fixation once the open repair is accomplished. Case Study is a case treated with metal plates, often called compression plating, because when they are properly applied, the plates force the bones together further improving stabilization and facilitating bony union.

Case Studies: Maxillofacial Fractures

A 30-year-old drug addict was unable to settle his financial differences with his supplier. The problem was settled with a 6-foot Douglas fir 2″ × 4″. A Panorex displays the damage (Fig. 7.14). The mandible is like a ring or circle (the circle is completed by the skull). When a ring fractures, it frequently does so in two places. To illustrate this, try to break a doughnut in only one place. This cannot be done—the doughnut always breaks in two places. The same is true with the mandible. In more than 50% of cases, there will be two or more fractures. This patient had two fractures, one on each mandibular body. Both fractures go through the root of a molar tooth. Because these fractures were unstable, the involved teeth were pulled. The right body fracture was reduced and held in place with a compression plate. The left body fracture was explored, reduced, and then wired into place. Insufficient dentition existed for arch bars to be used. The teeth were simply wired together as well as could be done. Postreduction films from this patient are shown in Figure 7.14B. The teeth were left wired in oc-

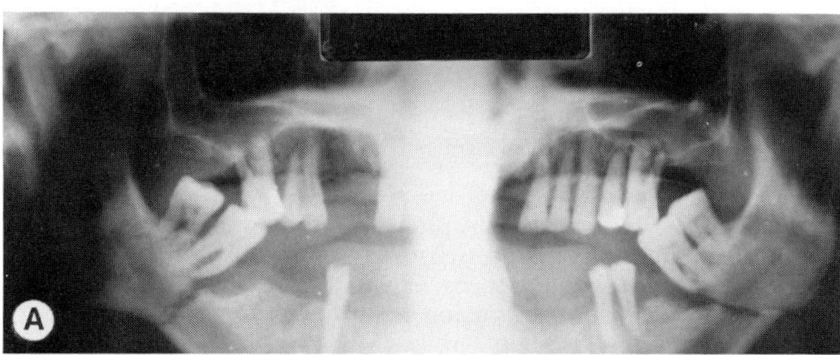

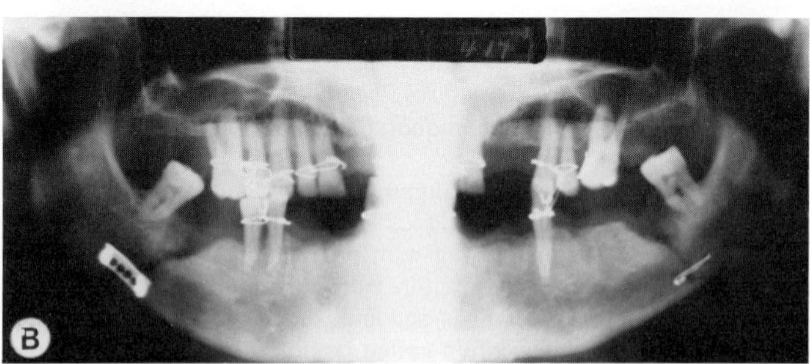

Figure 7.14.   Panorex of a 30-year-old patient with a fractured mandible. (A) Initial Panorex. (B) Postreduction Panorex.

clusion for 6 weeks and then the wires were removed. The fractures healed uneventfully.

A 65-year-old destitute male alcoholic was stumbling about when he was mugged. He suffered a fracture to both left and right mandibular bodies. The Panorex is shown in Figure 7.15A. The patient is edentulous, but he did have dentures. The right body fracture was displaced and required an open reduction and internal fixation with wire. The dentures were fixed to the mandible with circummandibular wires and to the maxilla with wires passing around the zygomatic arches. Arch bars were fixed to the dentures with fast-drying acrylic and the dentures were joined with rubber bands. The postreduction Panorex is shown in Figure 7.15B. This treatment stabilized the fracture and the patient's mandible healed uneventfully.

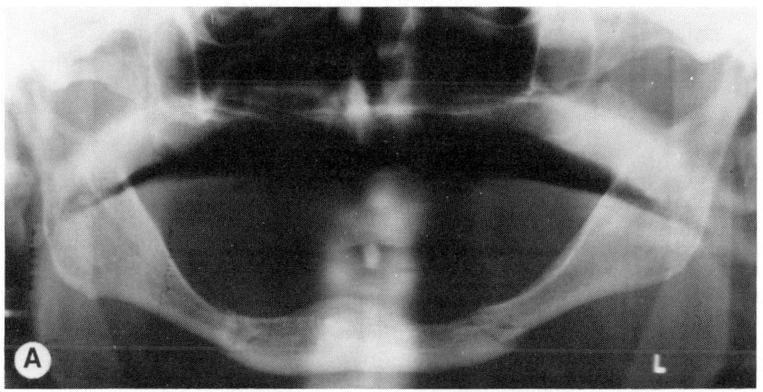

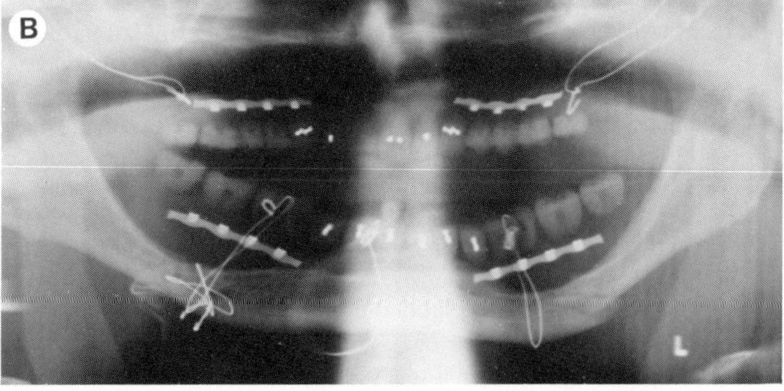

Figure 7.15. Panorex of a 65-year-old edentulous male with a fractured mandible. (A) Initial Panorex. (B) Postreduction Panorex.

This next case illustrates the use of the conventional X-ray examination of the mandible. A 40-year-old man was cheering for the Cincinnati Bengals against the San Diego Chargers while sitting in a bar in San Diego. A loyal Charger fan struck him viciously and he went out like a light. He was then brought to the emergency room. X rays from this patient are shown in Figure 7.16. A nondisplaced right angle fracture was seen. The patient, by this time sober and slightly paranoid about his safety in San Diego, flew home on the next plane and, hopefully, was treated in Cincinnati.

Case Study: Plating

Patient is a 19-year-old male who was sitting without a seat belt in the back of a sedan when the car was involved in an automobile accident at 60 mph. The patient lost consciousness for approximately 3 minutes and was transported by EMT to the trauma service at the UCSD Medical Center. The patient smelled of alcohol and on presentation at the Trauma Service was screaming in pain but was alert and oriented times 3. Vital signs in the field were BP 130/70, pulse 100, and respiratory rate 24. There was an obvious swelling with ecchymosis of the left side of the jaw. He was brought to the trauma unit and had a Glasgow Coma Scale of 14 (E4, V6, M6). He was at this time amnestic to the event and other than his head and neck, appeared to have suffered no major injury.

Examination of the head and neck revealed an obvious malocclusion. A mandibular fracture was present at the left angle to palpation. Right periorbital edema was present, periorbital ecchymosis was also evident. The extraocular movements were intact but the patient experienced diplopia on left upward gaze. He was tender to palpation over the left anterior maxilla and pain was also experienced when the palate was moved.

Plain films were taken and are shown in Figure 7.17. An obvious left mandibular angle fracture is seen. Facial fractures were not evident on the plain films, and a CT scan was ordered to better delineate the facial bones. These are seen in Figures 7.18 and 7.19 and show findings consistent with a LeFort I fracture. Both maxillary sinuses were fractured. The sinuses on one side were filled with blood and on the other side half filled with blood.

Once the patient was stabilized and the C-spine cleared, he was brought to the operating room and, under general anesthesia, arch bars were applied to the mandibular and maxillary teeth and interdental occlusion achieved with wires. The LeFort I maxillary fracture was approached through a sublabial incision

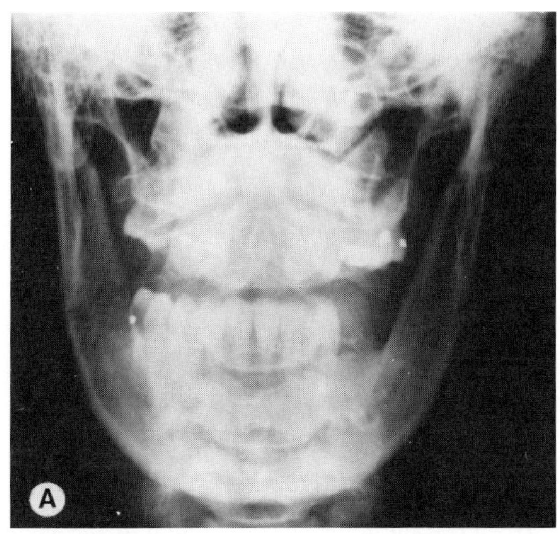

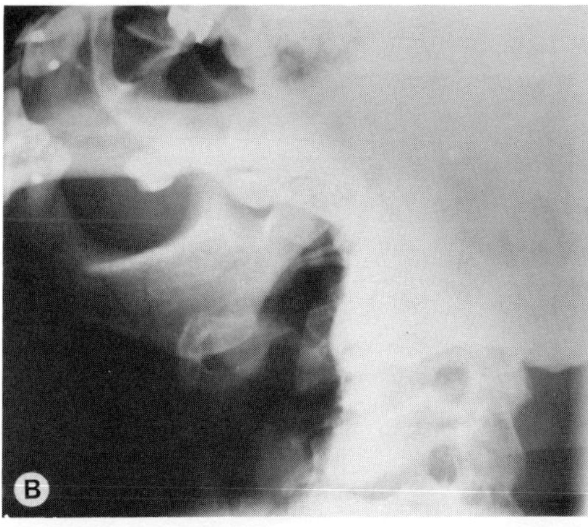

Figure 7.16.   X rays of a 40-year-old male with a fractured mandible. (A) PA view. (B) Right oblique view.

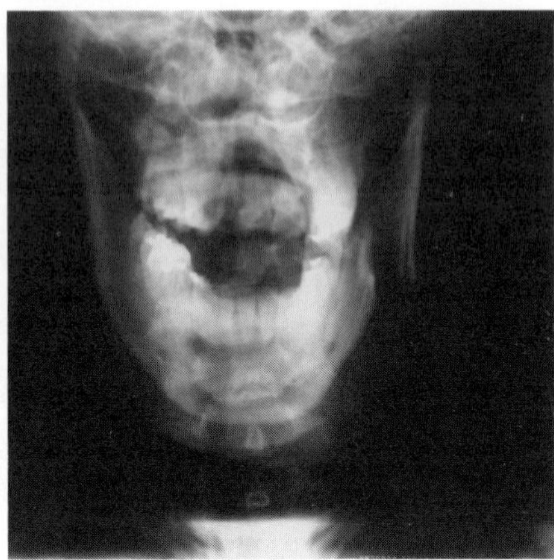

Figure 7.17.   Posterior/anterior mandibular X ray demonstrating widely diastased angle fracture.

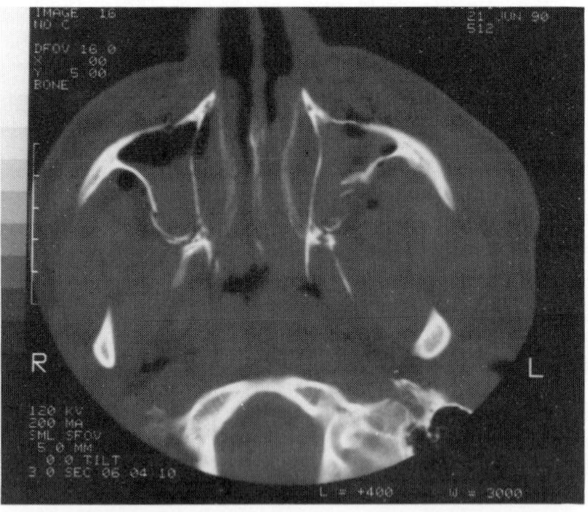

Figure 7.18.   Coronal CT scan through maxillary sinuses. Both maxillary bones fractured. Right maxillary sinus partially filled with blood. Air present immediately posterior and lateral to the sinus. Left maxillary sinus comminuted lateral wall. Sinus filled with blood. X ray findings consistent with a LeFort fracture.

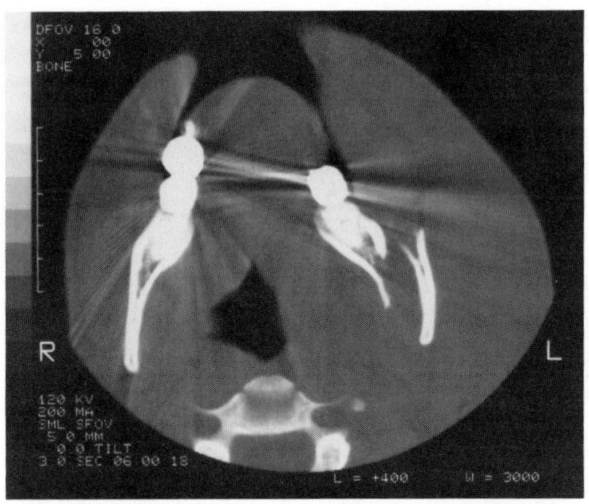

Figure 7.19. CT scan at the level of the mandibular angles. Left angle fracture with wide diastases clearly evident. Soft tissue swelling medially and laterally also seen.

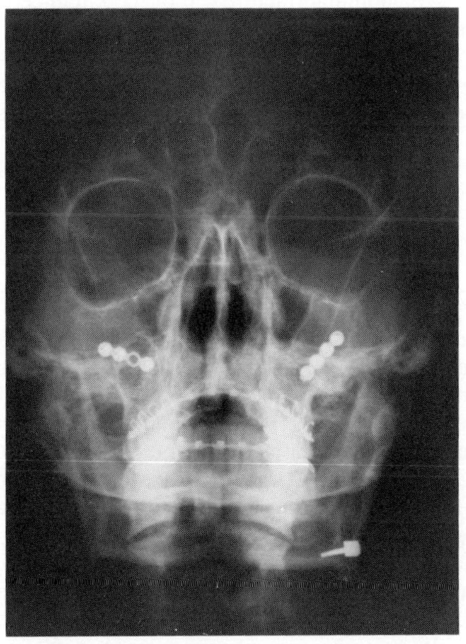

Figure 7.20. Postreduction plain film showing placement of metallic plates along the maxillary buttresses. Arch bars applied to maxillary and mandibular teeth. Plate wire and screws applied to left angle fracture. Bony alignment appears normal.

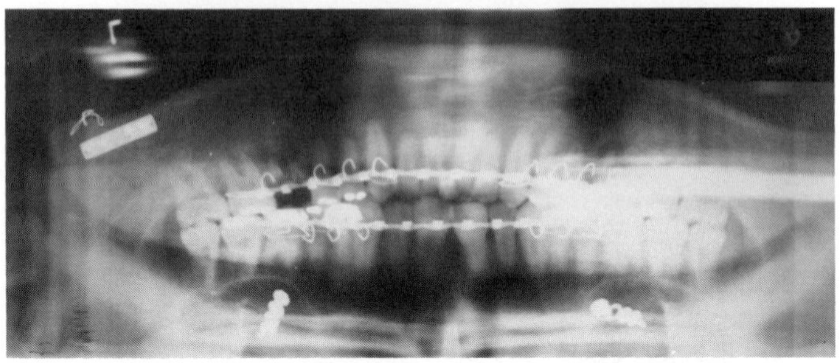

Figure 7.21. Postreduction panorex demonstrating plating of maxillary buttresses. Arch bars on maxillary and mandibular teeth. Plating and wiring of left angle fracture. Good anatomic alignment of left angle fracture.

and the two maxillary buttresses secured with metal plates and screws. The mandibular fracture was opened, reduced, and fixed with a plate and a stainless steel wire. The patient made an uneventful recovery. Figures 7.20 and 7.21 show the postreduction plain film and the postreduction panorex. The fractures are in good anatomic alignment. Common use of plates is shown both for the maxillary and the mandibular fractures. The arch bars are still in place, but will be removed in several days.

Trauma to Larynx and Trachea

Laryngeal and tracheal trauma requires an immediate consultation with head and neck surgery specialists. Hematomas, vocal cord paralysis, and laryngeal and tracheal fractures can all obstruct the airway instantaneously. If this occurs, the airway must be reestablished, either by an endotracheal intubation, by emergency cricothyrotomy, or by emergency tracheostomy. If the airway is not acutely obstructed, it should be evaluated. Appropriate instruments and personnel should be available in case an acute obstruction occurs.

Soft tissue X rays are sometimes useful for evaluating laryngotracheal trauma. CT scans are far superior and generally are much easier to interpret. For a very mild injury in which the physician has little reason clinically to suspect significant damage, soft tissue posteroanterior and lateral films should be ordered. If there is any suspicion that major injury has occurred and that significant fractures have been caused, the soft tissue films can be dispensed with and a CT scan obtained immediately.

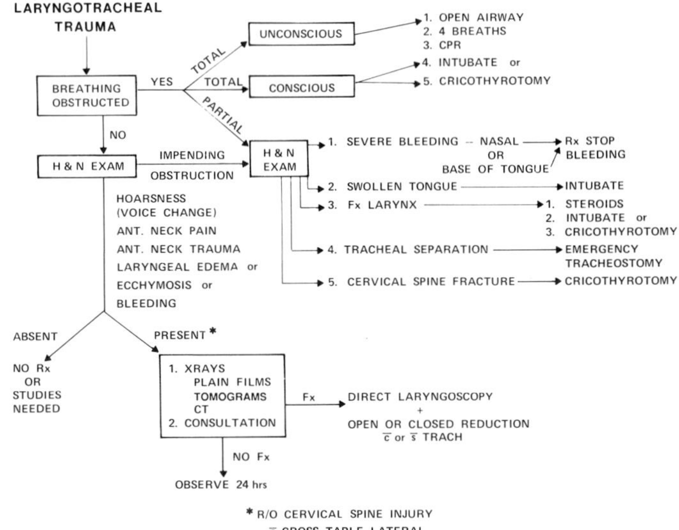

Figure 7.22. Assessment of laryngotracheal trauma. CT = computed tomography.

Whenever significant injury exists, direct laryngoscopy and bronchoscopy are indicated to better define the extent of the injury. A tracheostomy may be needed emergently to maintain the airway. Most fractures of the larynx and trachea require an open reduction. The bones may be wired together or simply stented and the airway generally protected with a tracheostomy.

Figure 7.22 is an algorithm for the evaluation of laryngotracheal trauma.

COSMETIC SURGERY

Cosmetic surgery has been performed for centuries, but it has recently become increasingly popular. Society's emphasis on appearance and youth is partly responsible for this explosive trend. Many physicians believe cosmetic surgery is vain and a waste of time and money. The patients benefited by those procedures feel differently, however. For many patients it has been a major turning point in their lives.

This kind of story occurs every day in facial plastic surgery. Society's standards are important to many people. Therefore, I am happy to be able to help this kind of patient in this manner. Each of you may have your own feelings and biases about plastic surgery, but you should reserve final judgement until you have met some of these patients and learned their feelings about their surgery. Independent of your own feelings about plastic surgery, some of your patients will desire this kind of surgery. Just as you would help a patient with peptic ulcer disease decide if he wanted abdominal surgery, you can help a patient decide if he or she wants cosmetic surgery. Just as you would refer the patient with peptic ulcer disease to a general surgeon skilled in abdominal surgery, you should refer the patient desiring cosmetic surgery to a head and neck surgeon skilled in cosmetic surgery. To provide some information on this topic, each of the common procedures is discussed separately.

Protruding Ears

Having protruding ears is not an easy problem for a child to handle; sometimes a youngster is called "Dumbo" and is asked if he or she can fly. The social pressures on a young child with protruding ears can at times be overwhelming. Otoplasty is a simple operation that pulls the ears back to a more normal position. This operation is best done just before children start nursery school. Children with protruding ears are very self-conscious and will often voice their desire for this surgery. Figure 7.23 shows a young man who wanted his ears fixed. He had always hated them, but had not known they could be improved. An otoplasty was performed.

Case Study: Cosmetic Surgery

One unforgettable case involves a 16-year-old girl who wanted a reduction rhinoplasty. She was neither gorgeous nor conspicuously unattractive. She did have a big nose. A rhinoplasty reduced and refined her nose. Everything healed well and she remained an average-looking girl, albeit with a smaller, more refined nose.

She returned to my office about 6 months after surgery. Her mother mentioned that prior to her nasal surgery this girl had never been out on a date. Now she had been selected to be the Queen of the Junior Prom. She was booked for dates 2 months in advance. To all appearances nothing had changed that much, even with the rhinoplasty. But the way the girl felt about herself had changed. She now carried herself with more assurance. She acted differently, and her classmates perceived her differently. The rhinoplasty was not physically responsible for this girl's change, but it made her feel better about herself. She had opened up psychologically and had become socially successful.

Rhinoplasty

Rhinoplasty is performed to remove bumps, fill in depressions, straighten the crooked nose, refine a bulbous, broad nose, and improve breathing. It should not be done until the patient has stopped growing,

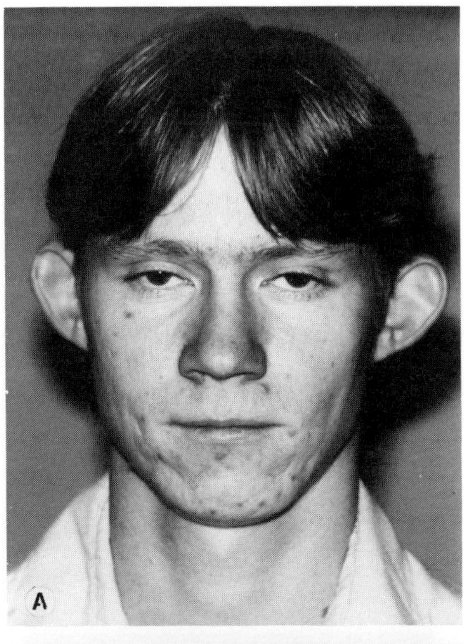

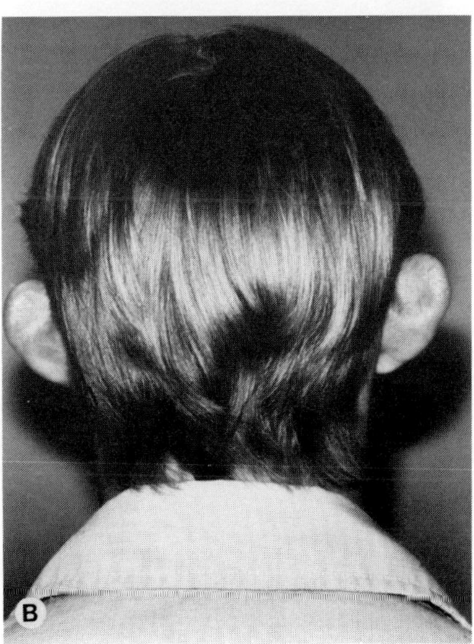

Figure 7.23. Patient with protruding ears, scheduled for oto-plasty. (A) Preoperative frontal view. (B) Preoperative posterior view. *(Continued on p. 196.)*

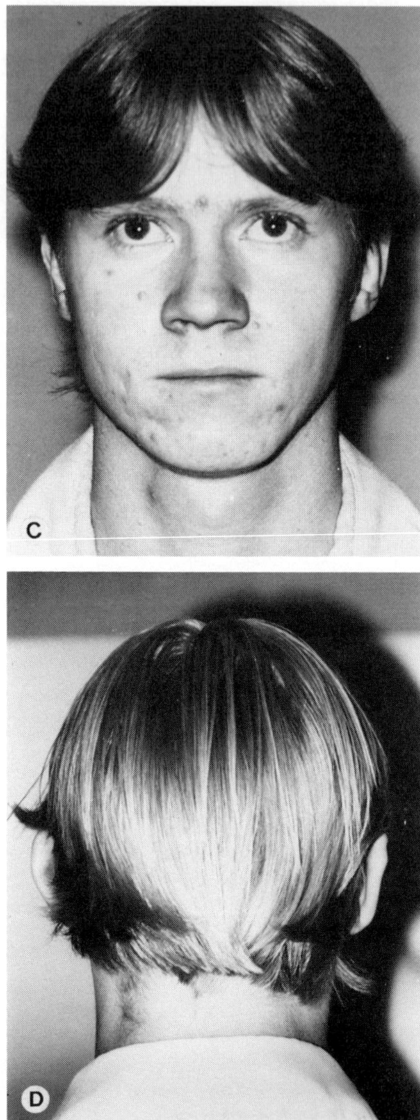

Figure 7.23.   (continued) (C) Postoperative frontal view. (D) Postoperative posterior view.

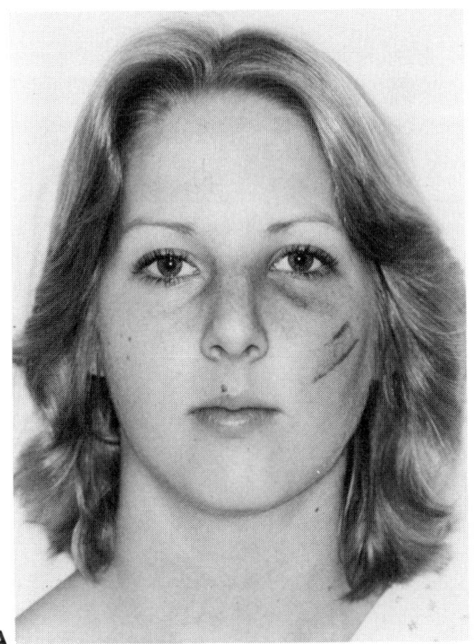

A

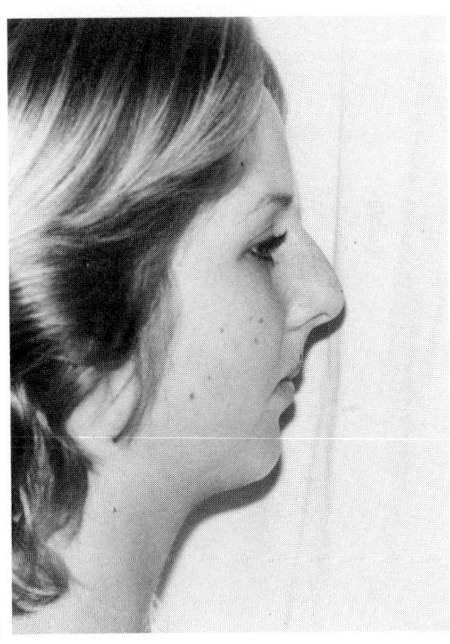

B

Figure 7.24. Preoperative photographs of a 16-year-old girl scheduled for cosmetic rhinoplasty. (A) Frontal view. (B) Lateral view.

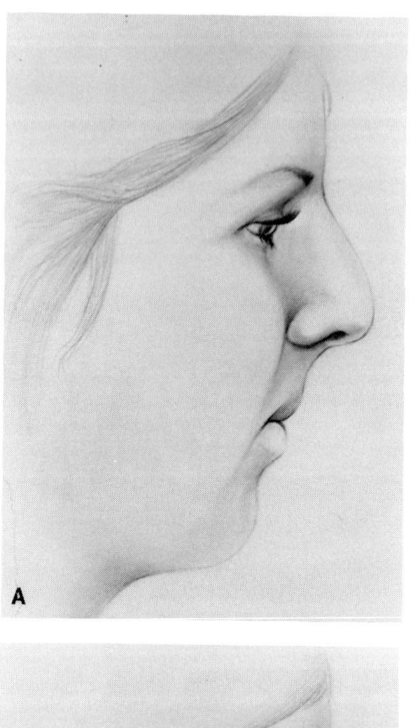

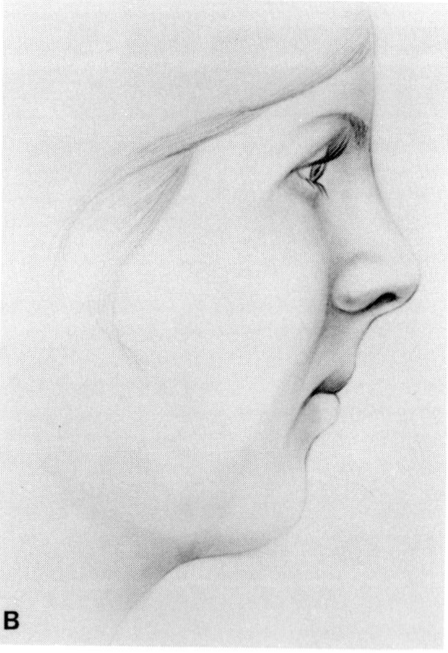

Figure 7.25. Rhinoplasty profile drawings of the same patient as in Figure 7.24. (A) Preoperative appearance. (B) Prospective drawing of nose as it might look after correction. *(Continued on p. 199.)*

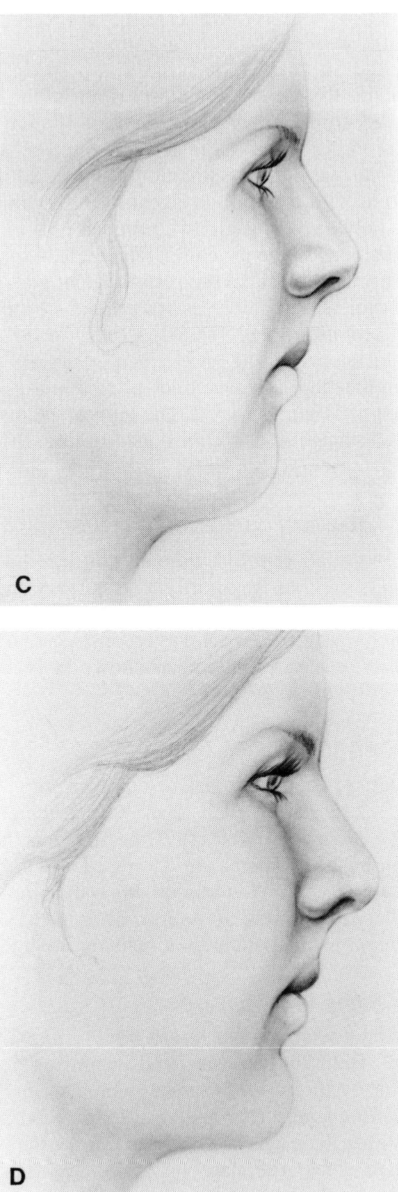

Figure 7.25. **(continued)** (C) Same profile as in (B), but with the nasofrontal angle better defined. (D) Same profile as in (B) plus an augmentation of the chin.

usually around age 16 years. The surgery is performed through incisions placed inside the nose. Rhinoplasty is one of the most complex facial plastic procedures. When done well, it is gratifying to both patient and surgeon. Crooked noses are straightened by rhinoplasty. Septal deviation causing nasal obstruction is corrected by septoplasty or, in combination with external changes, by septorhinoplasty.

Figure 7.24 shows a young girl who requested a cosmetic rhinoplasty. The patient was stable psychologically. Her expectations were reasonable. To better understand the planning that goes into this kind of surgery, the patient's profile was traced and is shown in Figure 7.25. Chin augmentation, (Fig. 7.25D) is easy to do and is an important part of facial evaluation and surgery. Surgery on the chin is frequently recommended as an adjunct to rhinoplasty. Figure 7.26 shows the patient following surgery. The biggest change is the shape of the nose. The change in the chin enhances the difference in the appearance of the nose.

Rhinoplasty and Reconstruction

Figure 7.27 shows a 30-year-old woman who had had a reduction rhinoplasty 5 years previously. Shortly after surgery she hit her nose on a cupboard. The nose became infected and healed, which resulted in the loss of the nasal bridge. This was reconstructed by augmenting the nose with a nylon mesh implant, as shown in Figure 7.28. The result is shown in Figure 7.29.

Cleft Lip and Cleft Palate

Patients with cleft lip and cleft palate deformity are evaluated by teams consisting of surgeon, pediatrician, speech therapist, audiologist, nutritionist, and social worker. These patients have multiple problems, and all of the problems are addressed as a combined effort by the palate team. Generally, the cleft lip is repaired at birth and the cleft palate between 18 and 36 months after birth. Care given by the cleft palate team to the patient continues into adulthood.

Surgery on the Aging Face

Surgery on the aging face is the most rapidly expanding field in cosmetic surgery. Both sun exposure and increasing age reduce the thickness and the elasticity of the skin, which wrinkles and sags. Several regions of the face can be analyzed for corrective surgery and treated. Forehead lift, face lift, and neck lift correct the drooping skin in these respective areas. Blepharoplasty restores the eyelids of an aging patient to a more youthful appearance. The nose lengthens as the patient ages and the chin often falls and recedes. These changes can be corrected by rhinoplasty and chin augmentation.

The very fine wrinkles particularly evident about the mouth and eyelids can be smoothed by using phenol or trichloroacetic acid (TCA) to cause peeling of the skin. This is called a chemical peel. It creates

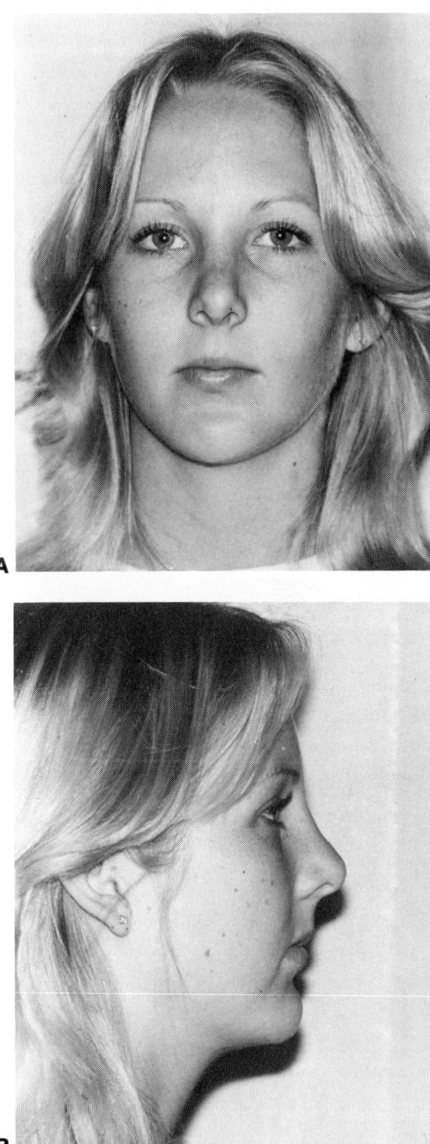

Figure 7.26. Postoperative photographs of patient shown in Figures 7.24 and 7.25. (A) Frontal view. (B) Lateral view.

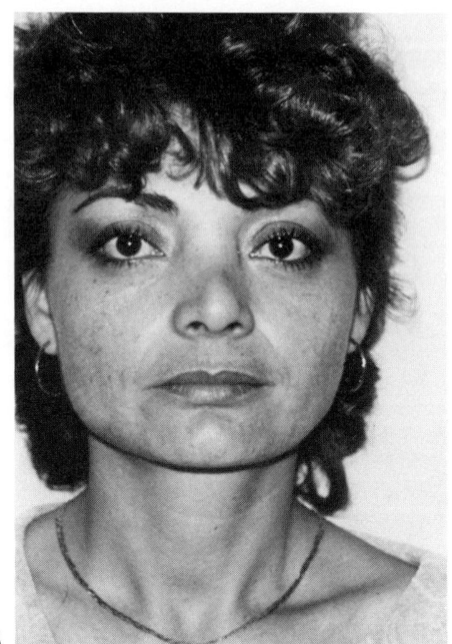

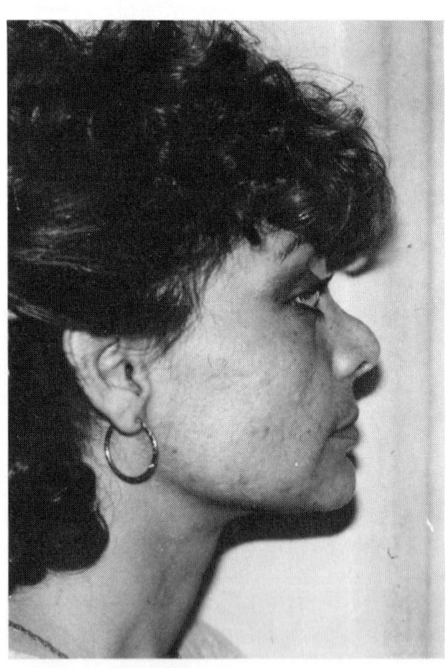

Figure 7.27. Preoperative photographs of a 30-year-old woman 5 years following reduction rhinoplasty and subsequent injury to the nose. A very obvious dorsal saddle deformity is evident. (A) Frontal view. (B) Lateral view.

a controlled second-degree burn. The resultant scarring tightens and smooths the skin surface. The same result can be achieved by sanding the face, a process called dermabrasion. Figure 7.30 shows preoperative and postoperative views of a middle-aged woman who wished facial surgery. Facial surgery to ameliorate the effects of aging is also commonly performed on men. Figure 7.31A shows a middle-aged man, who requested surgery. The surgery included a face lift, a blepharoplasty, and a brow lift. Figure 7.31B shows the result 10 months later. Notice the significant change in his eyes as well as in his neck. Figure 7.32A, shows a middle-aged woman with baggy and sagging eyelids, drooping nose, and hanging neck skin. There were many fine wrinkles around the patient's mouth. A blepharoplasty, face lift, rhinoplasty, and chemical peel were performed. The result, several months later, is shown in Figure 7.32B. A blepharoplasty was also performed on the woman shown in Figure 7.33. The young man

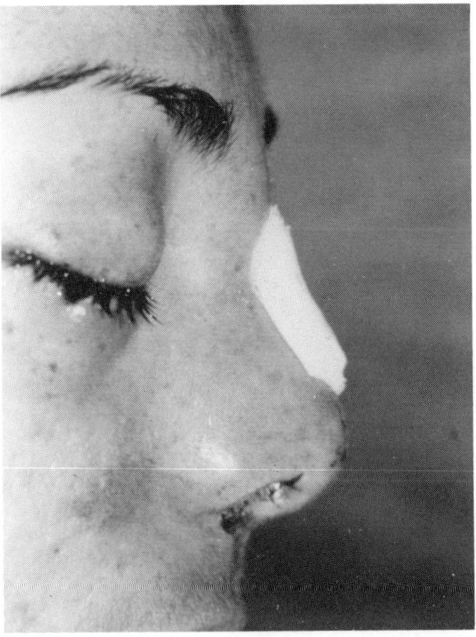

Figure 7.28. Intraoperative photograph of patient in Figure 7.27, showing the folded and trimmed nylon mesh graft placed over the dorsum just as it will be inserted.

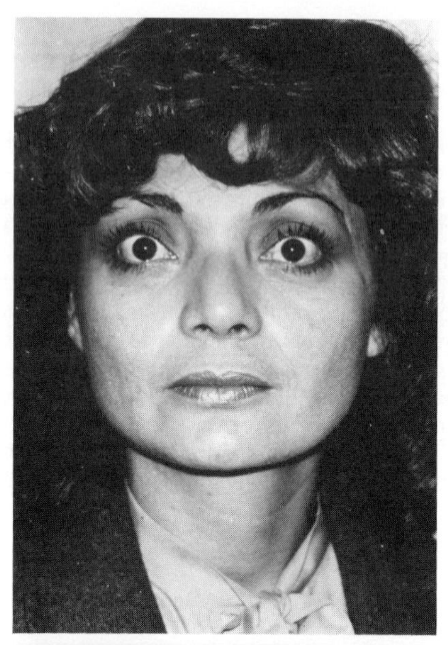
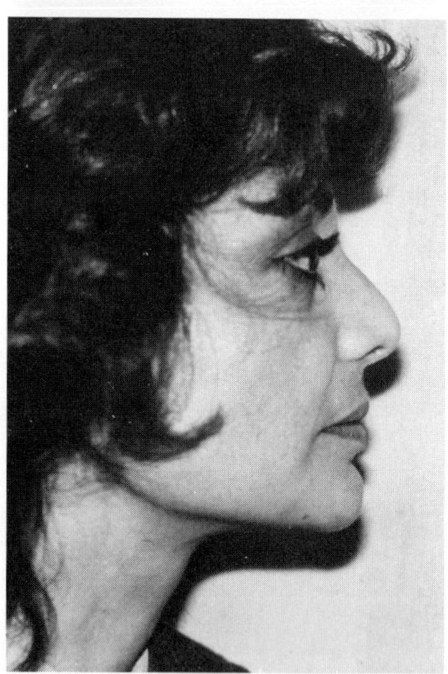

Figure 7.29. Photographs of patient in Figures 7.27 and 7.28, taken 10 months after rhinoplasty. (A) Frontal view. (B) Lateral view.

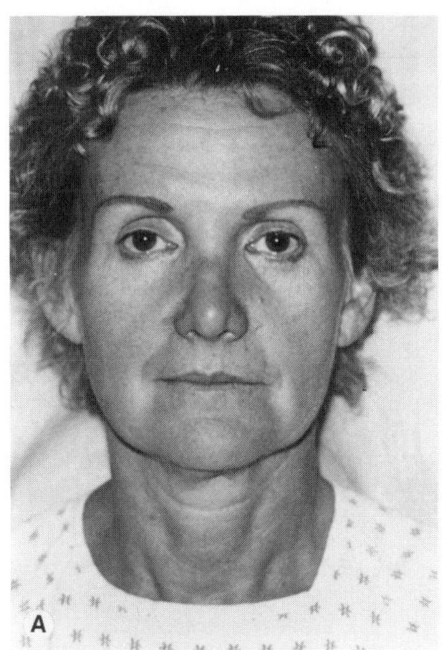
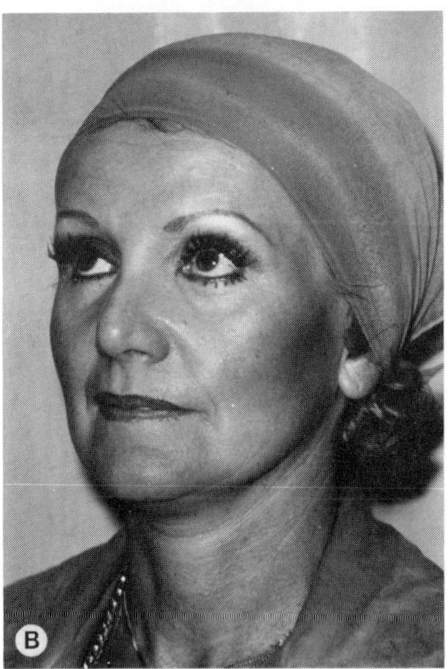

Figure 7.30. Face lift in a middle-aged woman who has already had a blepharoplasty and a rhinoplasty but wished to have the skin around her jaw and neck tightened. (A) Preoperative photograph. (B) Postoperative photograph.

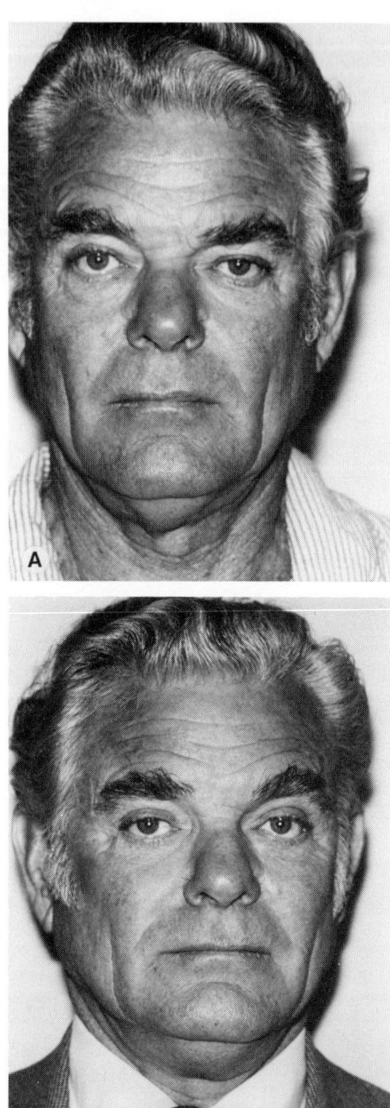

Figure 7.31. Middle-aged salesman who desired to look better for his work with people. A facelift, blepharoplasty, and browlift were performed. Postoperatively, his eyes are more open and appear more alert. The bags beneath his eyelids are gone, and the jowling and wrinkling in his neck are decreased. (A) Preoperative photograph. (B) Postoperative photograph.

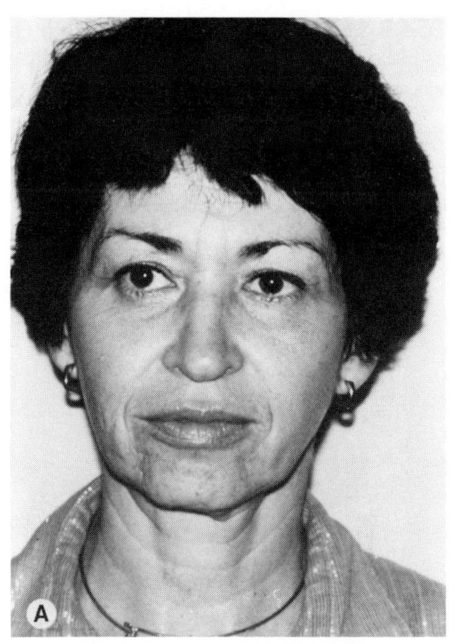

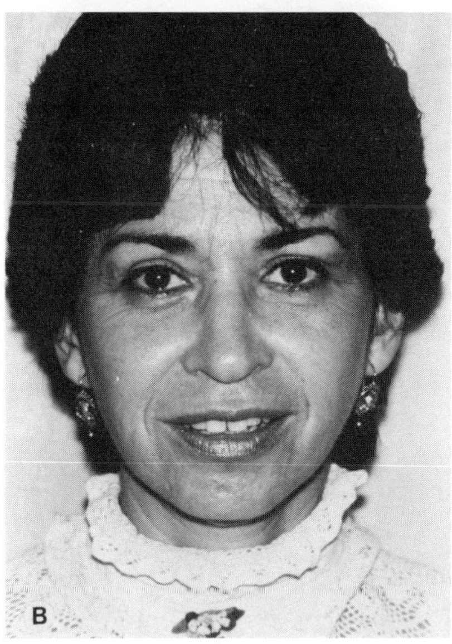

Figure 7.32. Facelift, blepharoplasty, rhinoplasty, chemical peel, in an elementary school teacher who wished to look younger for both professional and personal reasons. (A) Preoperative photograph. (B) Postoperative photograph.

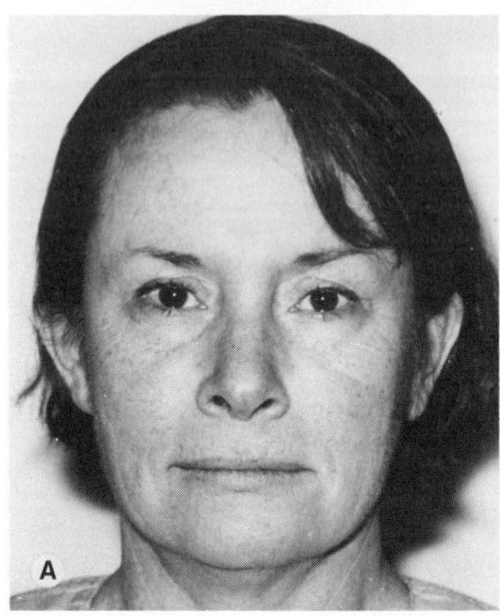

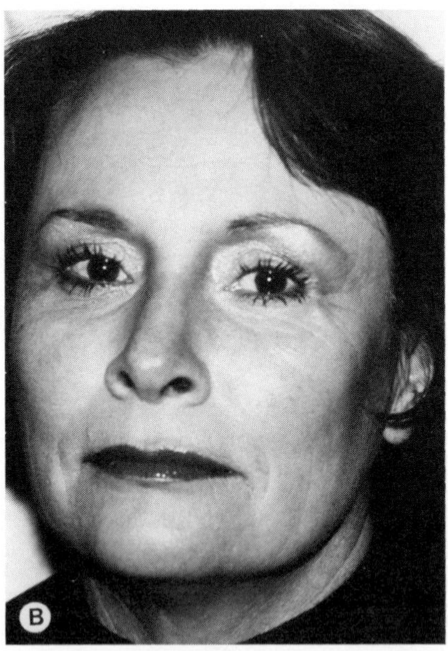

Figure 7.33.   A woman with drooping of the upper eyelids and a bagginess of the lower lids. A blepharoplasty was performed. (A) Preoperative photograph. (B) Postoperative photograph.

shown in Figure 7.34 was having difficulty obtaining work. He attributed this, in part, to his appearance, primarily his baggy eyelids. His face was somewhat featureless so in addition to blepharoplasty, he had implants to his cheek bones. He also had an augmentation mentoplasty (his chin was build forward). Both implants were hand-carved out of hard silicone. The improvement was dramatic. The patient improved his personal grooming and very quickly found a job.

Liposuction

Liposuction is widely used for cosmetic change. Originally developed to reduce the protruding female hip and the fat, saggy tummy, it is now used to remove fat throughout the body. It has proven useful in facial plastic surgery as well. Its greatest use is to remove fat in the submental region and to a lesser extent in the fatty, sagging jowl. In younger patients with elastic skin, liposuction is performed through a 5- to 6-mm submental stab incision. The liposucker is pushed through the subcutaneous tissues and when suction is applied removes the protruding subcutaneous fat. The skin contracts and a pleasing improvement can be achieved.

In older patients with greater skin laxity, liposuction alone will not provide the optimum result. Although the fat is easily removed, the skin does not contract and sagging facial and cervical skin is accentuated. For these individuals, face-lifting procedures are required. The two procedures are performed together, and superior results are achieved.

Liposuction is a contouring tool. It is not useful in the management of obesity.

Hair Transplants

Baldness can be corrected by placing hundreds of 4-mm, round punches of skin containing hair across the top of the head. These hair-bearing plugs are transplanted from the occipital hair-bearing scalp. More involved surgical procedures are also used, in which large flaps of hair can be transferred from the temporal region to the forehead. These techniques are more complex than those using hair plugs, but when they are successful, they create a much fuller, more natural head of hair.

Hair flaps are becoming increasingly used as surgeons and patients learn more about them. Figure 7.35 shows a man who was balding and did not like his appearance. A flap of hair measuring 4-cm wide and 28-cm long was raised from his right temporal and occipital region (Fig. 7.35B). This flap received its blood supply from the posterior branch of the superficial temporal artery. The flap was transposed to the front of his head and the 4-cm defect was closed. Three months later, the same procedure was performed on the opposite side. Several small finishing touches were applied and the final result is shown in Figure 7.35.C.

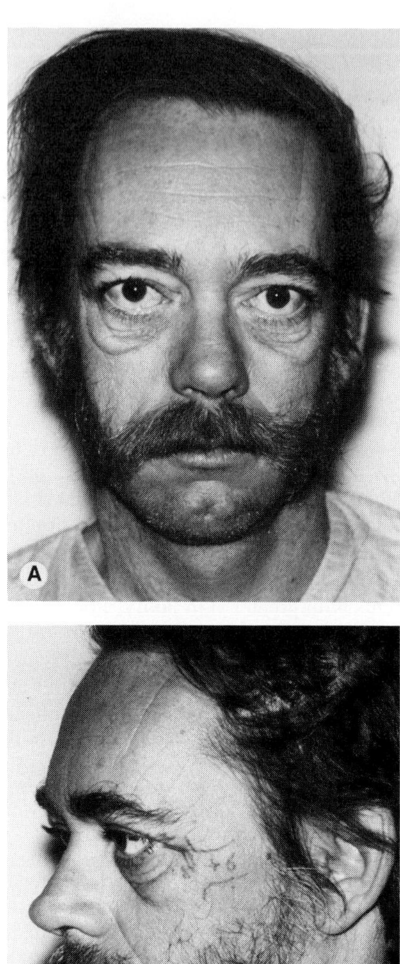

Figure 7.34. A patient with baggy eyelids, poor cheekbone definition, and a receding chin. Surgery (blepharoplasty, cheek bone and chin augmentation) improved all of these. (A) Preoperative photograph. (B) Preoperative photograph showing the area where the cheek bone implants will be placed. *(Continued on p. 211.)*

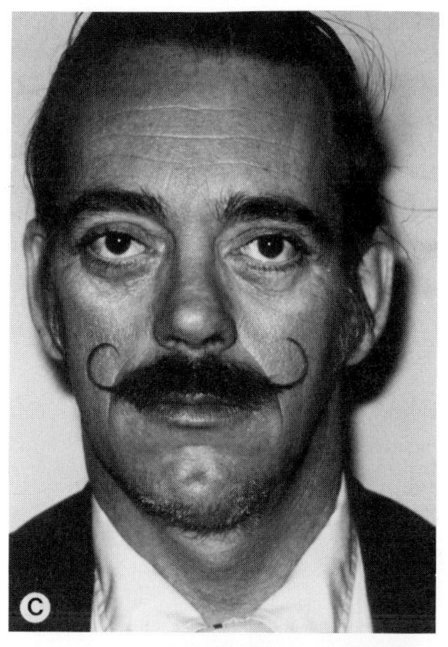

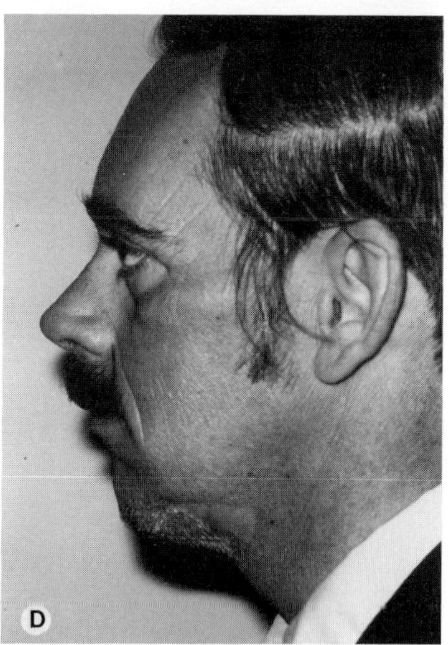

Figure 7.34. (continued) (C) and (D) Postoperative photographs.

211

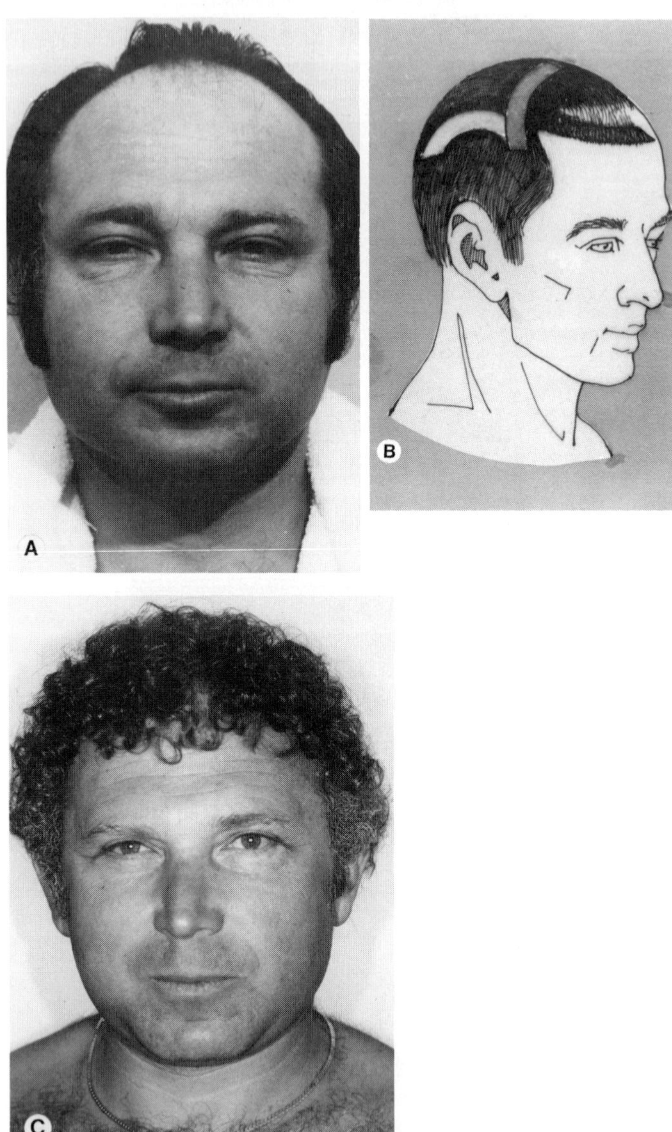

Figure 7.35. Hair-replacement surgery for a patient with male pattern baldness. (A) Preoperative photograph. (B) Drawing of a flap of hair transferred from the side of the head to the front. (C) Postoperative photograph. (Photographs courtesy of Drs. Toby Mayer and Richard Flemming.)

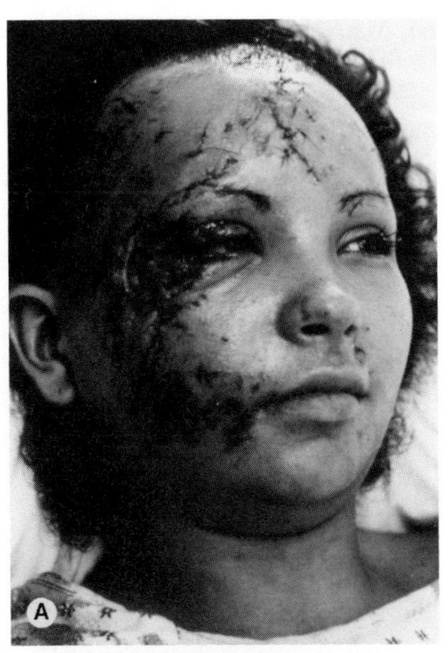

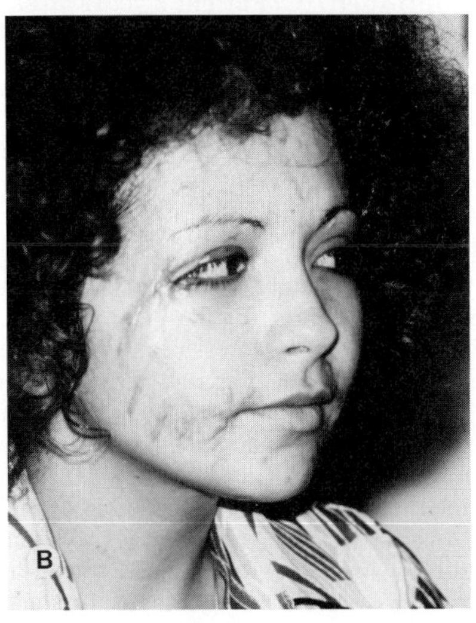

Figure 7.36. Scar revision in 18-year-old girl who was thrown from her automobile onto the pavement. She was placed in jail in Mexico and did not receive medical attention until 10 days after the accident. An attempt was made to remove all pieces of pavement from her wounds, but this was far from successful. (A) The patient as she presented to the University Hospital, San Diego. (B) Six months later, with heavy makeup camouflaging the tattooing and deep scarring. *(Continued on p. 214.)*

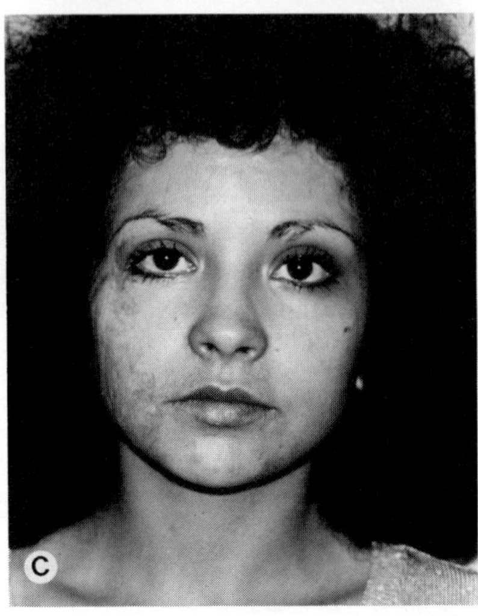

Figure 7.36. **(continued)** (C) Patient 2 years later, after several scar revisions, with no makeup. Notice that the tattooing is still not corrected. It never will be. Fortunately, makeup covers the deformity fairly well.

Other Surgical Procedures

A great variety of other cosmetic surgery procedures exist. Acne scarring is treated with surgery for the deep pits and injections of collagen to fill out remaining depressions. Facial scars are treated with excision, surgical camouflaging, and dermabrasion. Facial skeletal defects are filled in with custom-molded facial implants. The most striking facial surgery is that that repairs major congenital and developmental deformities. The entire facial skeleton can be lengthened, shortened, widened, or narrowed. The mandible or maxilla, or both, can be moved forward, backward, or sideways. All facial plastic and reconstructive surgery must be performed by well-trained, skilled surgeons. The patients must be psychologically stable. They must understand what is going to be done, what risks they are taking, and what reasonable goals they can hope to obtain.

Reconstructive Surgery

To me, the most challenging cases involve reconstruction after cancer surgery or trauma. Figure 7.36A shows a girl who was involved in an automobile accident while vacationing in Mexico. She reported she was not released by the authorities until the insurance issues were solved. We saw her for the first time 10 days after the accident. The wounds were cleaned as well as possible. Six months later, significant scarring and deformity persisted (Fig. 7.36B). Multiple scar revisions and dermabrasions were performed over the next year. Her appearance 2 years later is shown in Figure 7.36C. It is important to realize that this type of reconstructive surgery will never have a perfect outcome; its goals are improvement to the best degree possible. The patient must recognize these limitations. However, physicians must help patients heal psychologic wounds as surely as they help them heal physical wounds.

CHAPTER 8

AIDS and Otolaryngology

Otolaryngologists are involved with AIDS because 40% to 60% of AIDS patients present initially with disease in the head and neck, and therefore the otolaryngologist is required to suspect and diagnose the disease. Second, virtually all AIDS patients develop head and neck infections or tumors during their disease, and again the otolaryngologist is required to diagnose and assist in treatment.

AIDS is caused by a retrovirus, HIV-1. The enveloped virus contains a genomic-plus strand RNA; a DNA copy of the RNA is transcribed by the viral DNA polymerase or reverse transcriptase. Integration of the viral DNA into the host cell genome is necessary to establish infection. The integrated viral DNA is provirus. This is transcribed into viral RNA, which can either be used for the virion genomic RNA or be used for messenger RNAs, which are translated into virion proteins. Because retroviruses are generally not lytic, infection tends to be permanent.

The incidence of AIDS in the United States is monitored by the Center for Disease Control (CDC). As of November 30, 1990, there were 157,525 cases of AIDS. The incubation period for adults from the time of infection to the onset of disease is variable. The mean latency, according to 1988 CDC data, is estimated at 8 years for adults and somewhere between 1 and 3 years for neonates. It is estimated that there are between 750,000 to 1 million Americans already infected, and the number continues to grow. Advances in therapy are significantly prolonging the time from diagnosis of AIDS to death. Currently, the predicted mortality of AIDS is nearly 100%. The incidence of new cases is shown in Table 8.1.

A study by the US government published in 1988 estimates the cost of caring for a patient with AIDS at $57,000. Monies spent in 1988 for AIDS medical care was $2.2 billion; $4.5 billion is projected for 1991. Total national health care for 1991 is projected at $650 billion, almost 13% of the Gross National Product. The cost of AIDS

Table 8.1 New Cases of AIDS

YEAR	PATIENTS (N)
1983	2,852
1984	5,762
1985	10,598
1986	16,646
1987	22,680
1988	32,196
1989	35,238

medical care is less than 1% of our total health care expenditures. The cost of cancer is approximately 7% or $45.5 billion.

Seventy percent of AIDS patients are homosexual or bisexual males and 7% of these are IV drug users; 21% of the AIDS patients are heterosexual IV drug users. Only 2% to 3% of AIDS cases are associated with contaminated infusion-blood products. A small but increasing percent are neonates who acquire the HIV-1 vertically from an infected mother. The large majority of these women are IV drug users. The perinatal transmission rate is estimated at 30%. Approximately 80% of children with AIDS acquired it from infected mothers (70% of these are IV drug related, the remaining 30% are drug-product related). The neonatal transmission continues to increase, whereas the blood-product infection rate is decreasing.

The HIV-1 retrovirus infects T lymphocytes. These are called CD_4 lymphocytes. A normal, healthy person has approximately 1000 CD_4 lymphocytes per cubic milliliter of blood. When the CD_4 count drops below about 200 cells/mL, the body's immunity is significantly compromised, cellular immunity is affected predominately and, hence, organisms such as protozoans (Pneumocystis), fungi (Candida), and viruses (cytomegalovirus, herpes, and Epstein–Barr) that are normally cytotoxically killed by CD_4 lymphocytes, can and do produce disease. Tumors that are also under the surveillance of the CD_4 lymphocytes may begin to appear. Humoral antibody is also adversely affected, but not to the same degree as the cytotoxic immune system.

As the immune system is impaired, infections and tumors manifest. The opportunistic pathogens and the tumors are most notable for two reasons. First, these require cellular immunity that is now compromised. Second, current medicines against these opportunistic diseases have not been well developed, because prior to AIDS these were infrequently troublesome diseases.

The more common bacterial infections are still more frequent. They are of less concern for two reasons. First, humoral immunologic protection is not as severely affected and, second, current antibiotic availability provides excellent coverage to control and eradicate the bacterial disease.

Mycobacteria, particularly *M. tuberculosis* is a relatively common infection. It can present as a cervical adenopathy that may or may not have a pulmonary component. Extrapulmonary tuberculosis is particularly increased. The adenopathy is multiple. Normally, it is successfully eradicated with aggressive medical therapy, but if the nodes are large and develop necrotic foci, excision of the involved nodes is required. Atypical mycobacterial infection, especially M1 avium complex, are more common problems than *M. tuberculosis* in AIDS.

Fungi present frequently as a pathogen. Candida is certainly the most common and oral candidiasis is prevalent. Different presentations are seen. The patient will complain of a sensitive, painful mouth. On examination, the mucosa can be red and sensitive or there may be a build-up of white exudate. The candida can spread to the pharynx and esophagus and present as odynophagia. Treatment is topical clotrimazole. A 10-mg troche is prescribed five times a day, and success is dependent on the patient sucking the troche and keeping the clotrimazole in contact with the fungi as long as possible. The dissolved clotrimazole is swallowed, killing the candida in the pharynx and esophagus. Ketoconazole or fluconazole are alternatives for cases refractory to topical treatment. Histoplasmosis may present with ulcerative granulomatous lesions in the pharynx. Cases of disseminated histoplasmosis and coccidiomycosis are increasingly recognized.

Protozoans are uncommon pathogens in healthy humans. *Pneumocystis carinii* is an opportunistic protozoan and is common in AIDS. The vast majority of *P carinii* infections are pulmonary, but the protozoan has been reported in the external auditory canal, middle ear, thyroid, and in widely disseminated forms.

Viral infection is also common, and most of the viruses have head and neck manifestations. The most commonly recognized viruses include cytomegalovirus, Herpes simplex, Herpes zoster, Epstein–Barr, and human papilloma virus. These can be quite troublesome but are treated the same as in the general population. Ganciclovir is an important new antiviral licensed for treated of cytomegalovirus infection.

Lymphoproliferative head and neck disorders are also common and can be the initial AIDS presentation. Patients come to the head and neck surgeon for biopsy with a differential diagnosis including lymphoma, tuberculosis, and metastatic malignancy. Although a good history should identify important risk factors, the patient may not always provide the necessary information. HIV serology should be included in the initial work-up. Operating room and laboratory personnel must be warned that HIV is a consideration. Even in the AIDS patients, different lymphoproliferative disorders are seen. These include reactive lymph adenopathy, lymphoma, and metastatic malignancy.

Kaposi's sarcoma is also common in AIDS. Although it normally presents initially with mucocutaneous lesions, it can manifest in the cervical lymph nodes. In a patient with known AIDS, cervical lymph node biopsy is frequently requested to differentiate between the myriad of the aforementioned diseases. Special precautions are necessary for these surgeries and will be discussed later in this chapter.

There has been a tendency to subcategorize AIDS in the head and neck. For the most part, the diseases such as otitis media, tonsillitis, and sinusitis present the same and are treated the same as in patients who are immunologically normal. Opportunistic infections are similar to those seen in other immunocompromised patients. Perhaps these infections are more difficult to treat and, as with oral candidiasis, may require a longer medical regimen.

The only unique disease is Kaposi's sarcoma and when this presents in the mucosa of the upper aerodigestive tract, a biopsy to differentiate it from epidermoid carcinoma and necrotic infection is required.

For the most part, the otolaryngologist's primary role is to diagnose. The infections and tumors are often difficult for the primary care physician to diagnose, and biopsies of mucosal and lymphoid tissues can be helpful in keeping individual patients well. Because the otolaryngologist will see AIDS patients—some with a known diagnosis, some without—knowledge of the transmission risks is important.

Precautions to protect the entire health team are also important. Since the early 1980s, health care providers have feared (at times irrationally) contracting AIDS in part because of the social stigma and in part because of the prolonged, miserable death. To date, at least 18 health care providers have contracted AIDS by direct inoculation of blood; some were by needle stick with contaminated blood, fewer by spillage of blood into an open wound. Three cases involved spilling contaminated blood onto mucous membranes.

Current data indicate the risk of contracting AIDS from a percutaneous inoculation of infected blood to be 0.36%, or a little less than 1 in 250. The risk from mucous membrane contamination is so low that reliable statistics do not exist. The risk in the dental profession is estimated at 0.08% (1 in 1300) and occurs from spillage of blood-contaminated saliva into an open wound.

Although other body fluids—tears, saliva, peritoneal fluid, contain HIV, disease transmission has not been documented. The bottom line is that there may be a risk, but it is small.

Hepatitis B (HBV), on the other hand, is highly contagious. The CDC estimates that of 12,000 health care providers exposed annually to HBV, 500 to 600 require hospitalization and up to 1200 will become carriers; up to 250 will die annually as a direct result of HBV infection.

It therefore behooves all health care providers to take appropriate precautions. The following are the guidelines recommended by the Operating Room Committee at the San Diego Veteran's Administration Medical Center.

PREVENTION OF TRANSMISSION
OF AIDS AND HEPATITIS
FOR THE OR PERSONNEL

The OR Committee recommends that the Medical Center assume an active role in the prevention of transmission of AIDS and hepatitis for the OR personnel.

1. The OR Committee strongly supports HIV testing for all patients cared for at the Medical Center.
2. The OR Committee strongly supports the availability of AZT in the OR suite for immediate administration to consenting OR personnel accidentally incurring percutaneous or mucous membrane exposure to blood or body fluids.
3. All OR personnel should be tested and immunized for HBV.
4. The OR Committee strongly supports HIV transmission precautions for all OR personnel.
   a. The following patient categories are recognized:

   High risk = known HIV or HBV positive or at high risk for HIV or HBV infection;

   Low risk = known HIV and HBV negative or at low risk for HIV and HBV infection.

   b. The patient category will be determined by the most senior surgeon in the OR.
   c. The following operational policies are recommended:

Attire	High Risk Patients	Low Risk Patients
Eye protection	Required	Required
Double gloves	Required	Optional
Impermeable gown	Required	Optional
Boots	Optional	Optional
Air filter system	Optional	Optional
Techniques		
Intra-Op self gowning	Required	Required
Post-Op hand washing	Required	Required
Sharps isolation	Required	Optional
Student/intern exclusion	Required	Optional

   d. The following clarifications are noteworthy:
      (1) Eye protection or a face shield is required for the entire operating team at all times. The only exceptions are in-

dividuals performing surgery through a microscope or endoscope where such gear compromises visual acuity. Where high-pressure irrigation is used the operating team will be required to wear full face shields during the irrigation.

(2) Heavy orthopedic gloves may substitute for double gloves. Double gloves or heavy gloves are recommended for all operating team members at all times. Exceptions are those procedures requiring the delicate touch offered by single gloves.

(3) Impermeable gowns are recommended for all cases where excessive blood loss, high volume irrigation, or extensive splattering is anticipated.

(4) Impermeable boots are recommended for cases involving blood or fluid spillage beyond the operative field.

(5) Air-filter systems are expensive and should not be used routinely. However, high risk cases involving extensive splashing, plumes, or aerosolization make air-filter systems a serious consideration.

(6) Following the initial incision, surgeons scrubbing into a case must gown and glove themselves if the scrub nurse has contacted tissue, blood, or body fluids directly or by handling instruments.

(7) All OR personnel are required to wash their hands immediately after degloving.

(8) Special techniques for passing sharp instruments, pins, and wires will be required in all high-risk cases.

(9) Inexperienced personnel such as interns and medical students are not permitted to scrub on high risk cases.

Although it is acceptable for medical students to work with and examine AIDS patients, the inexperienced should not:

1. Draw blood on HIV- and HBV-positive patients.
2. Assist at surgery on HIV-positive patients.
3. Perform surgery on HIV- and HBV-positive patients.

Until venepuncture and surgical skills are developed to a high level of proficiency, the risk is simply unnecessary.

Every health care provider should be vaccinated against HBV infection. Last, should an inadvertent blood inoculation occur, particularly from a known HIV-infected patient, everyone should have made the decision to take or not to take Zidovudine (AZT) treatment. If one has opted to take AZT, it should be readily available and should be taken within 1 to 5 minutes of the inoculation.

CHAPTER 9

Psychosocial Considerations

The preceding chapters have focused primarily on the physical complaints and the clinical findings in the diseases under discussion, but these make up only a portion of the total picture. Each patient is an individual with a unique and complex psychosocial background. The physician who takes the time to develop good rapport with the patient, learn the patient's psychosocial history, and then discover how this history interacts with the patient's current complaints will be a better diagnostician and a more effective healer. There are several compelling reasons for a physician to be skilled in the psychosocial side of medicine. First, the physician who establishes rapport and expresses a real interest in the patient will obtain a far more accurate history. The patient senses this interest and is more likely to relate an accurate history, even if it contains embarrassing elements. I remember a patient referred to the gastrointestinal service with abdominal cramping and diarrhea. She had been fully evaluated previously at two well-known medical centers. None of the examiners had made a definitive diagnosis. She was again evaluated extensively, but no diagnosis was apparent. I was an intern at this time and had devoted a great deal of time and effort in establishing rapport with this patient. After 2 weeks of asking about her psychosocial history, she finally trusted me sufficiently to tell me about her disastrous marriage. She knew it was the cause of her diarrhea. Once we knew her real problem, therapy was directed at her personal life and not toward correcting a colon disorder. However, it required rapport to obtain the correct history and to make the correct diagnosis. Only then could appropriate therapeutic recommendations be made.

Second, a disease causes certain symptoms. The patient interprets and expresses these symptoms. This interpretation and expression accounts for at least 50% of the disease process and has significant bearing on therapeutic success. The physician who takes psychosocial history, understands the patient, and uses this information effectively will be a far more effective healer. A good example of the way psychologic factors may work is provided by the common viral head cold. If you develop a cold on a day when you have a final examination in biochemistry, for example, the cold will make you miserable and you may not be able to take the test. But if you catch it on a day when you are packing to go home for an exciting vacation, the cold may hardly be noticed. Patients with diseases such as sinusitis, headache, allergic rhinitis, neck ache, backache, dizziness, and tinnitus all express different degrees of discomfort and incapacity from the disorder. It is not only the variability in disease severity that causes this discrepancy but also the patient's psychosocial situation and attitudes. Pain tolerance is another good example. If you hit your finger with a hammer on an otherwise good day, the pain is intense immediately but dissipates rapidly. However, if you and your domestic partner are having a disagreement and out of anger your partner hits your finger with a hammer, the pain will be intense and will last as long as you wish to make it last. Patients are just the same. To be an effective healer, their psychosocial situations must be understood as well as how the current disease interacts with their lives.

Third, some diseases are purely psychosomatic. These must be recognized and dealt with accordingly. Migraine headache is a good example. It is clear that migraine is tension related. Many physicians, however, treat migraine as if it were a physiologic disease. To me, it makes more sense to discover the patient's stresses and tensions and try to direct therapy at improving these problems. If you are not totally successful treating the patient's stresses, it is fine to treat the pain additionally with drugs intended to decrease the discomfort. Another example of a psychosomatic illness is a patient with a neurosis, such as depression, who has physical symptoms. The astute physician will recognize the depression and refer the patient for psychiatric help. The physician who fails to obtain a psychosocial history may admit the patient to a hospital with the diagnosis of "malaise and weight loss," then order a complete work-up to rule out cancer. When the evaluation is negative the patient will be discharged and told that he or she is "fine." This kind of error occurs daily with physicians who do not take the time and make the effort to understand the patient's full medical and psychosocial history.

Finally, medicine can be a rewarding experience for a sensitive, caring physician. If you allow yourself to learn about and understand your patients, a far more important relationship will develop; the physician may benefit as much as the patient. Many physicians take the time to know their patients. People frequently ask "What happened to the good old country doctor?" Although we answer that medicine has become too sophisticated and is now practiced in hospitals with MRI, CT scanners, computers, and similar equipment, this is not really answering the question. What the patients miss is the doctor who took the time to talk to patients and to understand them as individuals. Many physicians today still spend time learning about their patients. For these patients and physicians, a very special and rewarding relationship develops.

A multitude of texts have been written that cover the psychosocial sciences ad infinitum and ad nauseum. I do not wish to contribute to the nausea, but I would like to illustrate some of my comments with several case examples.

CASE EXAMPLES

The first patient was a third-year medical student who stopped by my office and asked me if I would look at his sore throat. The ensuing conversation went as follows:

Q. Tell me a little about your sore throat.
A. What would you like to know?
Q. When did it start?
A. It started 2 to 3 weeks ago and has been fairly constant since then.
Q. Have you had any fever or malaise?
A. No.
Q. Any lymph node swelling in your neck?
A. No.
Q. Any other symptoms?
A. No.

At this point I looked at the patient's throat, which was entirely normal. There were no abnormal swellings in his neck. Based on the history and lack of physical findings, it was my opinion that there was no readily apparent physical basis for his complaint. I therefore explored his psychosocial history.

Q. What are you doing these days?
A. I am on Surgery at the Navy Hospital.
Q. How is that?
A. Pretty good. We are very busy and I am working very hard. There are two patients with osteosarcomas, one of the leg and the other of the arm. In addition, we have several patients with metastatic terminal cancers.
Q. I have a feeling, from the way you talk, that these cases are upsetting you.
A. Yeah, I guess so. None of the surgeons seem to spend time with these patients. The patients have no family— no nothing—and so I have been spending a lot of time with them. We begin rounds at 6:30 each morning and don't finish until midnight.

Q. Has anyone helped you with your feelings about the pa-
tients with cancer?
A. No, all the doctors just avoid the patients and the subject.
Q. So you have to fill in for them?
A. I guess so.
Q. Let me back up to your sore throat for a minute. What
is the pain like? Is it a stabbing pain, a burning pain, or
more like a tightening?
A. It is a tightening or a constricting pain.
Q. Do you think this might be related to your feelings about
the patients on the Surgery Service?

The student smiled at this point, as he, too, had made the
obvious connection between the sore throat and the cancer patients. We then went on to talk about his feelings and how he
could learn to deal with them.

This student was a healthy, psychologically well-adjusted
individual. He was not neurotic or psychotic. The stress of his
life had become acutely overwhelming, and he had no outlet
for his tension. He developed some spasms in the muscles in
his throat. These spasms caused pain and became a focus for
his attention. Discovering and talking about his real problem
relieved some of his stress and the physical symptoms rapidly
disappeared.

I do not want to suggest that all patients with a straightforward, acute, short-term medical illness need a complete psychosocial history. You should be sensitive to the patient whose
complaints are not classic. The patient just described had complaints that were extremely atypical for a sore throat. A short
psychosocial history uncovered the patient's real problem. Throat
cultures, antistreptolysin O titers, complete blood cell count,
sedimentation rate, chest X ray, skin tests, penicillin, acetaminophen, aspirin, and even codeine would all have been
costly and ineffective.

The next patient was a 45-year-old male who smoked and
drank heavily; he presented with a chief complaint of sore throat
of 3-weeks duration. History revealed 54 pack years (2 packs/day
for 27 years) of smoking, heavy alcohol use, and a recent 10-
lb weight loss. Examination revealed a very reddened pharyngeal mucosa, but no evidence of infection or tumor. The patient
was reassured that nothing was wrong. He was advised to stop
smoking and drinking.

Two weeks later, he returned with the same complaints. He
stated he had decreased his smoking to one pack per day and

was only drinking three highballs at night. Physical examination was unchanged. A throat culture was taken and a chest X ray was ordered. He was given a prescription for antibiotics for a 2-week period.

The patient returned again 4 weeks later. His symptoms had abated on the penicillin, but had recurred soon after stopping the medication. Examination was unchanged. Again he was advised to stop smoking and drinking. He was given a prescription for viscous lidocaine and instructed to return in 1 month. He returned 6 weeks later with his throat condition virtually unchanged. Diagnosis was a mucosal irritation from the smoking and drinking. The patient was advised that his problem would not go away until he stopped smoking and drinking.

I was aware that I did not enjoy talking to this man. I did not relate well to him and, although I felt it my responsibility to rule out infections and tumors, I did not wish to spend time on his psychosocial history. Much to my dismay, he kept returning to me—sometimes better, sometimes worse. I even suggested he see a different doctor, but he felt I knew him and should continue to treat him.

After a year of this, I finally decided to find out more about this man. His father had died a painful death of cancer of the throat. His mother had died an alcoholic. At the age of 16 years, he was left to care for three brothers and two sisters. He dropped out of high school to do this. He worked his way up in a small business and was now relatively successful.

He had married at the age of 25 years and had two children. His wife had left him 1 year ago, and he was now living with his 18-year-old son. The son did not work and was heavily into drugs. The patient's only support group was his friends at a local club, where they drank and smoked together. He was very alone, and very frightened that he, too, would die of cancer of the throat. He and I discussed all of this and how it affected his throat symptoms. With my urging and his approval, he entered a therapy group available through the hospital.

I saw him 6 months later for an ear infection. He was still smoking but had stopped drinking. He was seeing his wife and they were considering moving back together. His throat was still sore, but he knew that was related to his smoking. It did not bother him as much as it had previously.

This is an example of a real physical complaint whose perception is greatly enhanced by the patients' psychosocial situation. I failed to deal with this effectively, and the symptoms persisted. When I finally explored his psychosocial history, I was able to direct this man to psychologic help. This greatly improved his life and decreased his sore throat.

The next patient was a 35-year-old woman who came to my office for revision rhinoplasty. All her life she had wanted the size of her nose reduced and finally had sought consultation with a plastic surgeon. He told her there was "nothing to it," and the surgery was performed. The result 6 months later was unchanged from the preoperative appearance. A second procedure was carried out, and postoperatively the nose developed a serious, unsightly dorsal depression. A third procedure corrected this. The nose was now less attractive than originally, and the patient was very unhappy. A fourth procedure was recommended.

At this point, the patient had lost trust in the original surgeon and had sought a second opinion. On examination, the skin of the patient's nose was found to extremely thick. The patient desired a refined, delicate tip. In an effort to achieve this result, the surgeon had removed virtually all of the lower lateral alar cartilages. There now was just a blob of skin held up by the patient's septum. The surgeon had made a serious error in even trying to produce a refined tip on a patient with such thick skin. The patient's goals were virtually unobtainable.

The patient's desires were still the same—namely, for a refined, delicate tip to the nose. She had always hated her nose and now she hated it even more. She could not be happy until her nose was fixed. She had decided to go from surgeon to surgeon until she found one who could solve her problem.

I then asked her about her personal life. She was unmarried and worked as a business administrator for a large firm. She had been dating the president of that firm. The relationship had not progressed, and she was disheartened by that. Her plastic surgeon was a customer of the same firm, which further complicated her life. She was therefore considering moving to a new city and taking a new job.

We talked for a long time and I explained the following to her: First, the type of nose she wanted was not possible to create. No matter how many surgeons she sought, she would never acquire a refined nose. Furthermore, she had a wide, full face. A thin, refined nose would not even look good, as it would be out of balance with the rest of her face. I felt that she was using her nose in part as a scapegoat for some of her other problems, and I made the following remarks: "First, you are pretty just the way you are. You don't need a different nose. In any case, there is nothing you can do to get a different nose. It is not possible. You must stop looking for nasal surgery. Accept what you have, take care with your appearance, and you will look just fine. Face your other problems for what they are. Do not displace them onto your face. Running away will not solve them."

We talked about all this for some time, and then she left. Two months later she telephoned me. She said that she had thought a lot about our conversation. She realized and accepted that her nose could not be changed, and so there was no use in worrying about it further. She faced her problems and now felt better about herself. She felt good about her work and felt settled about her life.

This is a prevalent problem in all areas of medicine and is particularly common in the field of cosmetic surgery. A patient has a personal problem, either at work or at home. Rather than facing that problem, the patient focuses on some real, slight, or even nonexistent physical problem or deformity for which correction is sought. An astute physician should recognize this when only a slight or nonexistent physical deformity or disorder is present. It is far more difficult to recognize the underlying psychologic problem when the patient focuses on a very real physical deformity. A patient may just as easily focus on a problem such as complaints of sinus symptoms. As physicians, we must fully evaluate each patient. When there is psychologic pain, we must recognize this. Psychologic pain cannot be cured by treating a physical illness, and in these cases we must first diagnose the problem and then direct the therapy appropriately.

A 56-year-old woman was referred to me to rule out sinus causes for headaches. Her history is long and is summarized briefly here. The patient was well until 10 years prior to this consultation, when she began having headaches on the left side of her head. She took aspirin for these, but over the years the headaches had slowly increased in intensity. The patient saw her family physician on occasion and he told her they were just nerves and prescribed diazepam and aspirin. About a year ago, the headaches became so severe she consulted another physician, who obtained a complete history and physical examination. He ordered a complete battery of blood tests. He also concluded it was just nerves, but told the patient that if she wished further examination she should consult a neurologist. At first she hesitated to do this, but the headaches were becoming unbearable. The neurologist obtained a complete history and physical examination and then ordered a skull series, electroencephalography, and CT scan. He concluded that she had atypical migraine and prescribed an ergotrate. This made the patient quite dizzy, but did not alleviate the headaches. He then tried propranolal hydrochloride. This too failed to cure the headaches. He then sent the patient to a surgeon for a temporal artery biopsy. In the preoperative evaluation she was found to have a guaiac-positive stool specimen. An upper and lower gastrointestinal tract study was ordered. The patient also had a sigmoidoscopy and a gynecologic consultation. All these yielded negative results and she finally had the temporal artery biopsy. The results were nondiagnostic. By this time, her medical bill had reached $9000 and she still had headaches. She was advised to seek psychiatric consultation.

Instead, she returned to her family physician, who suggested she consult first with an opthalmologist to rule out eye problems and with a head and neck surgeon to rule out sinus problems. The opthalmic consultation was negative.

She next came to see me. After obtaining the history just described, I asked her where it hurt and she pointed to the side of the head. The head and neck examination was normal. Pressure over the temporomandibular joint elicited some tenderness, which radiated up to the side of the head. Her teeth were ground down due to bruxism.

Her psychosocial history revealed that her husband had had a heart attack 10 years earlier and had retired. He now sat around the house, and she spent her whole day caring for him. His retirement and disability checks were not entirely sufficient and so they had to watch their money carefully. This patient felt miserable. As she put it, she just gritted her teeth and did the best she could. She had always ground her teeth in response to stress and over the past years had been doing it more and more.

I made the diagnosis of temporomandibular joint pain resulting from bruxism. I explained the mechanism of this disorder to the patient. I referred her to a dentist to have a plate made for her to wear at night and sent her to a Crisis Center for help with her home situation.

I received follow-up letters from the dentist and the psychiatrist. The patient's symptoms had greatly decreased with the bite plate, which she wore at night and through much of the day. The Crisis Center employed a home visiting nurse who visited the couple, and the husband now was learning to care, in part, for himself. The patient had joined a therapy group. She was now working during the day and was feeling much better about herself.

It is interesting to note that in this case, several physicians had made the diagnosis of nerves but none had effectively communicated to the patient the cause and mechanisms of her pain nor had they helped the patient to deal with her stresses. Had her original physician done so, he might have saved this patient years of unnecessary suffering. He would have also saved society at least $9000 in medical bills.

Many physicians would tell you cases like these are uncommon; they would state that all patients have problems, but that the medical diseases they bring to their physicians are real problems and are not linked, as I suggested, to their personal lives. I disagree. Although half of the patients I see have a disease unrelated to their psychosocial history, my interest in their personal lives enhances our relationship and their trust in me as a physician. The other half of the patients I see do have a disease intimately connected to, if not directly caused by, their psychosocial situations. For these patients, taking a psychosocial history and responding appropriately is a critical or crucial aspect in diagnosing their disease and in prescribing appropriate treatment.

Mr. G. was a 70-year-old man who developed an epidermoid carcinoma of the palate. This was treated with radiation therapy, recurred, and was treated with cryotherapy. About this time, he developed multiple cranial nerve deficits. Extensive evaluation failed to identify any cause. It was suspected that he had metastatic tumor to the base of the skull. After 6 months of progressive agony, repeat CT scans and tomography documented the existence of metastatic disease.

It had been the belief of all the physicians treating this man that some central nervous system lesion must exist, but we had been unable to demonstrate it. For these reasons, we worked with the family intensively toward an ultimate cure. When the tomograms finally showed the destruction at the base of the skull, it was clear that cure was not possible.

The evening before he died, I spent 2 hours talking with his family. After a lot of soul-searching, the family members all agreed that they did not wish to prolong Mr. G.'s agony. We discussed autopsy and funeral plans. The family lived 120 miles away. They asked me when he might die and I replied that I didn't know—it could be tonight or next week. I told them they had been tremendously supportive for Mr. G. and had done everything possible to help him. They should not feel guilty if he died peacefully when they were not there. They had been present and helpful in his lifetime. In fact, sometimes patients do not die until the family leaves. It is almost as if they hold on for the family. Once alone, they can let go.

The family accepted this and decided to drive home. Mr. G. died in his sleep that night. When I notified the family, I restated how supportive they had been and how kind it had been not to fight and prolong his agony. Two weeks later I received a card from the family thanking me for my kind care.

This case represents one of the most important functions we perform as physicians—helping not only the patient but also the family. When a person dies the family suffers, too. As a physician you can help them in their grieving. Family members frequently feel guilt. You can help them understand and deal with grief, guilt, and anger.

A 29 year old x-ray technician/instructor complained of a sore throat. On the small clinic desk, beside his brand new University Medical Center chart, was a 2-inch thick chart of records, copies of his medical care from a neighboring institution. I chose to disregard the chart and asked him what was wrong, wherein he replied he had a sore throat that had been going on for years. He mentioned he had brought with him the records of his evaluation and care and gestured to the chart on my desk. I had no idea how one could possibly generate a 2-inch chart for a sore throat. I asked him if I could read the chart to which he assented.

The chart was of particular interest for it began with copies of all of the bills generated for this sore throat; I quickly added up the various pages and came to a sum exceeding $10,000. The medical portion of the chart indicated that this individual had presented to a primary care physician with a complaint of a sore throat. The examination at that point indicated some mild pharyngeal inflammation. The diagnosis of pharyngitis was made, a culture was taken and the patient was prescribed penicillin. He reported no real change in his pharyngeal pain and a second antibiotic was prescribed, a little broader in its coverage and a little more expensive.

A note 2 weeks later indicated that the sore throat had not changed and a laboratory investigation was begun. The throat culture and initial sampling of blood failed to enlighten the treating physician. The patient was then referred to an ENT physician who performed a much more elaborate examination, found nothing, spoke of endoscopies and biopsies, mentioned smoker's pharyngitis and ultimately cultured the patients' throat and prescribed a new antibiotic. This too failed and hence a tonsillectomy was recommended and performed.

Following recovery from the tonsillectomy the sore throat persisted and a more rigorous laboratory examination was requested. Sinus x-rays were obtained as was a barium swallow. The radiographs were all interpreted as negative. The head and neck surgeon concluded that this was a psychiatric disturbance and referred the patient to an infectious disease consultant.

The infectious disease physician cultured the throat several times, skin tested both arms and when all results were normal again requested antibodies and titers to all known pathogens. The results from these all were read as negative or normal. Additional esoteric tests were ordered. Allergy/immunology consultation was obtained, desensitization was initiated, all to no avail.

I asked the patient to describe his sore throat which he described as a pain or soreness in the back of his throat, a fairly typical middle pharyngeal muscle spasm. It was a pain that hurt with each swallow but did not feel like a lump in the throat. At no time had he felt systemically ill and there was no history of fever, sweats or any other symptoms commonly associated with infectious illnesses.

I asked the patient about the stresses in his life; he questioned how I could consider a stress-related problem when I had not even looked at his throat. I asked him if he would like me to look at his throat and he responded that he would. I performed a very careful head and neck examination, all of which were entirely within normal limits.

I again asked him about the stresses in his life and commented, "you have been through one of the most elaborate, expensive workups for a sore throat I have ever had opportunity to read. You have had every test I have ever known for a sore throat, including many I have never known. You have had a constant sore throat for a period exceeding 1 year. It has been unresponsive to most of the medications known to affect disorders of the throat. Your symptoms have remained unchanged for an entire year and you have a completely normal examination." The patient replied, "I was always worried that it was going to turn out to be stress related. Where do I go from here?" I responded that he would need to obtain a psychiatric evaluation and that he and the psychiatrist could explore these matters.

Each physician had at one time entertained a diagnosis of a mental health illness, none had communicated this as a possibility to the patient. The patient had exhausted the physicians, the laboratories and himself and so self-referred to the university.

The following is a summary of the psychiatrists's evaluation. The psychiatric diagnosis would be best categorized as

Axis I: 1. Psychogenic pain (sensory conversion)
            2. Dysthymia (depressive neurosis)

Axis II: Mixed compulsive, passive dependant personality.

Axis III: Sore throat (functional)

Axis IV: Stress factors: intrapsychic solely.

Axis V: GAF = 58.

The patient was initially highly resistant to any form of psychotherapy. After much working through the history it emerged that this young man was the oldest son of a high-school principal father who consciously decided to make this son the model young man in his community. All of the son's choices were made for him with no input from him. The patient had a younger sister with whom he felt a significant bond but shared no emotional intimacy. The patient also felt dominated by his mother. The patient still phoned his father weekly and sought his advice on all aspects of his life.

The patient was treated with modified short-term therapy, focusing on the present and the relationship between the patient and the psychiatrist. The psychiatrist pointed out the patient's subtle ways of avoiding emotional contact with him. During the challenge phase of his resistances he redeveloped the acute pain in his throat (severe motor tension caused by compulsive inhibition of aggressive impulses) whenever he wanted to verbally lash out at the psychiatrist.

The treatment did not go smoothly. The patient frequently wanted to terminate. However, he began seeing a woman and began a romantic relationship. The phone calls to his father decreased and he began to make his own decisions. He grew fond of the psychiatrist and related his feelings in a spontaneous way. The students in his class saw the most profound change. They previously taunted him relentlessly, and he was incapable of standing up for himself. One day he broke out in a rage at them and insisted on proper respect and decorum in his classroom.

The psychiatrist's summary of the psychodynamics involved is as follows. The patient's sense of self was damaged by his parent's need to control him. He was not allowed to separate, individuate, rebel and make his own mistakes. He suffered from enormous castration (retaliatory) anxiety from all authority and peer figures so his only answer to his perceived dilemma was to appear cooperative but to passively rebel by both withholding and sabotaging his own life. The meaning of the sore throat is complex. The patient was appearing to the medical profession because he was in pain and he was hoping (and frightened) that some physician would recognize the true source of his pain. At the same time as each clinician missed the actual cause of his suffering he took great delight in retaliating secretly by castrating the clinician through his own treatment-resistant symptoms.

This kind of sadomasochistic patient is extremely common in medical and surgical practice and is frequently misdiagnosed and mistreated at great expense to the patient, the profession, and society.

Appendix: Head and Neck Surgery Study Outline

This appendix is an outline developed for the head and neck surgery medical rotation at the University of California at San Diego. It is included here for the reader's use.

I. EAR
  A. Auricular hematoma
    1. Treatment: drainage
       a. Fine needle aspiration
       b. Incision with or without drain (rubber band)
       c. Pressure dressing
  B. Foreign body in the external auditory canal
    1. Treatment: remove gently—if not easy, perform with microscopic control with general mask anesthesia
  C. Otitis externa
    1. Symptoms
       a. Pain
       b. Itching
       c. Decreased hearing
    2. Signs
       a. Auricular pain (elicited by shaking auricle)
       b. Erythema of external auditory canal
       c. Edema of external auditory canal
       d. White keratinous debris in canal
    3. Etiology
       a. Prolonged water exposure
       b. Cotton swab or other foreign body trauma
    4. Organisms
       a. *Pseudomonas aeruginosa* (95%–99%)
       b. Fungal (<5%)

    5. Treatment
       a. Domeboro otic (aluminum sulfate and calcium acetate) 30 ml bottle, 4 drops qid in affected ear or Cortisporin Otic® Solution (polymyxin B-neomycin-hydrocortisone), 10 ml bottle, 4 drops qid in affected ear
       b. For pain: aspirin, aspirin with codeine, or non-steroidal anti-inflammatory agents *and*
       c. Local heat application (e.g., heating pad)

D. Surfer's Ear (External Auditory Canal Exostoses)
    1. Symptoms
       a. Associated with prolonged, cold, salt water exposure; seen in surfers and professional divers
       b. usually present with otitis externa
    2. Signs: generally three exostoses seen in external auditory canal, often white, firm to palpation, adjacent to tympanic membrane
    3. Treatment: if occluding more than 50% of canal, surgical removal required

E. Acute Otitis Media
    1. Symptoms
       a. Fever
       b. Otalgia (pain)
       c. Decreased hearing
       d. Pressure in the ear
       e. Discharge only with perforation
    2. Signs
       a. Red, bulging tympanic membrane
       b. Conductive hearing loss—diagnose with tuning forks
    3. Treatment
       a. Adults: amoxicillin, 250 mg
         #30
         1 po tid
       b. Children 5 years old or under: amoxicillin, 40 mg/kg/d (3 doses daily for 10 days maximum)
    4. Follow-up: appointment in 10–14 days

F. Chronic Otitis Media
    1. Symptoms
       a. Chronic drainage, often foul-smelling
       b. Decreased hearing
    2. Signs—These are all signs of what is properly called cholesteatoma
       a. Foul-smelling drainage during periods of exacerbation

    b. Tympanic membrane perforation, often at the margin
    c. White keratinous debris
3. Treatment
    a. Cortisporin otic solution®, 10-ml bottle: 4 drops qid in affected ear *and* penicillin, 250 mg #60 1 po qid
    b. Surgery (when not infected): tympanomastoidectomy
4. Complications
    a. Brain abscess
    b. Meningitis
    c. Lateral sinus (sigmoid sinus) thrombosis
    d. Facial nerve paralysis
    e. Labyrinthitis

G. Serous Otitis Media
1. Symptoms
    a. Decreased hearing
    b. Feeling of fullness in ears
2. Signs
    a. Retracted tympanic membrane with no response or reverse movement on pneumomassage
    b. Conductive hearing loss: Can be measured with 256- and 512-cps tuning forks, audiometry, or tympanometry
3. Etiology
    a. Poor eustachian tube function
    b. Allergic upper respiratory tract disease
    c. Bacterial rhinosinusitis
    d. Residual otitis media
    e. Nasopharyngeal obstruction: adenoids, nasopharyngeal tumor
    f. Cleft palate
4. Treatment
    a. Observe for 2 weeks
    b. If no change, give decongestant-antihistamine combination for 2 weeks
    c. If no success, prescribe antibiotics (ampicilin, amoxicillin, or penicillin)
    d. If still no success, change to another decongestant and antihistamine for 2 weeks or a short course of systemic steroids
    e. If no success, observe for 2 weeks with no therapy
    f. If no change, myringotomy and insertion of middle ear ventilation tube should be performed by head and neck surgeon

- H. Otosclerosis
    1. Symptoms
        a. Hearing loss
        b. Tinnitus
    2. Signs
        a. Conductive hearing loss with normal otoscopy
        b. Audiogram: conductive hearing loss, sometimes combined with a sensorineural hearing loss
    3. Treatment: Stapedectomy
- I. Meniere's Disease
    1. Symptoms
        a. Fluctuating hearing loss
        b. Tinnitus
        c. Vertigo
        d. Feeling of fullness in the ear
    2. Signs
        a. Fluctuating hearing loss on audiograms
        b. Otherwise negative results on vertigo work-up
    3. Treatment
        a. Acute treatment for vertigo: see "Vertigo" (IV.E)
        b. If patient allergic, give treatment for allergy
        c. If disease is psychosomatic, advise psychiatric care
        d. Otherwise, trial of low-salt diet and diuretics, if this fails, prescribe diazepam—if diazepam fails, try promethazine hydrochloride or other phenothiazine
    4. Follow-up care by specialist in head and neck medicine and surgery
- J. Presbycusis
    1. Symptoms
        a. Decreased hearing
        b. Ringing in ears
    2. Signs: Sensorineural hearing loss on audiogram
    3. Treatment
        a. Rule out noise-induced hearing loss by history and audiogram
        b. Hearing aid if recommended by specialist in ear disease
- K. Acoustic Neuroma
    1. Symptoms
        a. Hearing loss or
        b. Vertigo or
        c. Facial paralysis
    2. Signs
        a. Sensorineural hearing loss with poor discrimination
        b. Abnormal BERA

c. Unilateral weakness on electronystagnography
d. MRI or CT scan indicating cerebellopontine angle tumor
3. Treatment: Refer to specialist in head and neck medicine and surgery
L. Temporomandibular Joint Syndrome (TMJ)
1. Symptoms
a. Patient complains of ear pain in which pain is anterior to ear canal; pain involves muscles innervated by CNV, particularly the muscles of mastication
b. Clicking in temporomandibular joint
2. Signs
a. Pain on finger pressure over joint when opening and closing mouth
b. Poor dental occlusion or loose-fitting dentures
c. Spasm of involved muscles
d. Anxious, depressed, or hysterical patient often shows bruxism and teeth clenching
3. Treatment
a. Treat psychosomatic aspects if cause is stress
b. Refer to general dentist or orthodontist with experience in TMJ and occlusal problems
c. Refer to TMJ clinic

II. OTALGIA WORK-UP
Rule out lesions by history and physical examination
A. External Auditory Canal
1. Auricular hematoma
2. Foreign body in the ear canal
3. Otitis externa
4. External auditory canal tumor
5. Otitis media—acute or chronic
B. Temporomandibular Joint
C. Referred Pain from Inflammatory or Neoplastic Lesion
Pain referred from
1. Nasopharynx
2. Tonsil
3. Base of tongue
4. Larynx
5. Pharynx and hypopharynx
Evaluate by examination, endoscopy cultures, and biopsies

III. HEARING LOSS DIFFERENTIAL DIAGNOSIS
A. External Auditory Canal Obstruction
1. Wax
2. Foreign body
3. Otitis externa

    4. Exostoses
    5. Tumor
  B. Middle Ear
    1. Acute otitis media
    2. Chronic otitis media
    3. Serous otitis media
    4. Tympanic membrane perforation
    5. Otosclerosis
    6. Ossicular discontinuity
    7. Round window rupture (barotrauma)
  C. Inner Ear
    1. Meniere's disease
    2. Presbycusis
    3. Noise-induced hearing loss
    4. Otosclerosis
  D. Central Nervous System
    1. Cerebrovascular accident
    2. Brain tumor
    3. Psychiatric disease

IV. VERTIGO WORK-UP
  A. History
    1. Vertigo
      a. Onset
      b. Intensity
      c. Duration
      d. Association with nausea and vomiting
    2. Hearing loss
    3. Tinnitus
    4. Feeling of fullness in ear
    5. History of ear pain, infection, surgery, and so forth
    6. Recent illness
    7. Current medications
  B. Examination
    1. Hearing (tuning fork)
    2. Otoscopic
    3. Ophthalmic, to include extraocular movements, examination for nystagus, and retinoscopy
    4. Cranial nerves, with particular attention to nerves 3,4,5, (especially corneal), 6,7,9, and 10
    5. Neck examination to recognize carotid artery disease
    6. Blood pressure, to consider hypertension and orthostatic changes
    7. Pulse, to diagnose arrhythmia
    8. Neurologic, to exclude neurologic disease, especially multiple sclerosis and cerebrovascular accident

C. Laboratory
1. Complete blood cell count to rule out anemia
2. Electrolytes determinations to detect any imbalance
3. Calcium determinations to detect hypocalcemia
4. Tetraiodothyronine to detect hypothyroidism
5. VDRL and FTA-ABS tests to rule out tertiary syphilis
6. Cholesterol and triglyceride determinations to detect hyperlipoproteinemia
7. Blood and urine tests for diabetes
8. Electrocardiography with rhythm strip to diagnose cardiac disease
9. Audiogram and tympanogram to evaluate hearing: if a loss exists, to evaluate type of loss
10. Brain stem-evoked-response audiometry
11. Electronystagmogram to test labyrinthine function, gaze nystagmus, response to caloric irrigation; extremely useful to identify labyrinthine disease and also helps localize lesions either in the labyrinth or in the central nervous system
12. Equitest—This is a balance test and separates vestibular cerebellar and peripheral causes of imbalance
13. MRI or, if unavailable, CT scan of the internal auditory canal to evaluate cerebellopontine angle tumors, particularly acoustic neuroma
14. Cervical spine series—the cervical spine is closely connected to the labyrinth via a vestibulospinal reflex arc. Cervical spine disease can cause vertigo and must be evaluated.

D. Differential Diagnosis: this is not intended as an exhaustive differential, but rather to provide some insight into the different diseases that can cause vertigo; with persistence a diagnosis can be made in over 90% of vertiginous patients
1. Otologic
    a. Acute otitis media
    b. Serous otitis media
    c. Chronic otitis media
    d. Perilymph fistula
        i.   Traumatic
        ii. Poststapedectomy
        iii. Barotrauma (round window rupture)
    e. Labyrinthitis
        i.   Bacterial
        ii. Viral
        iii. Toxic
    f. Meniere's disease
    g. Vestibular neuronitis

      h. Benign positional vertigo
      i. Acoustic neuroma or other cerebellopontine angle tumors
  2. Central nervous system
      a. Stroke
      b. Transient ischemia attacks
      c. Multiple sclerosis
      d. Neurosyphilis
      e. Meningitis or encephalitis
      f. Migraine
  3. Neck
      a. Osteoarthritis
      b. Carotid artery stenosis
      c. Vertebrobasillar artery insufficiency
      d. Subclavian steal syndrome
  4. Metabolic
      a. Hyperglycemia or hypoglycemia
      b. Hyperthyroidism or hypothyroidism
      c. Electrolyte imbalance
      d. Hypercalcemia
      e. Anemia
      f. Polycythemia
      g. Leukemia
  5. Infections
      a. Influenza
      b. Herpes zoster
      c. Measles
      d. Mumps
      e. Other viral illness
  6. Drugs
      a. Streptomycin
      b. Kanamycin
      c. Gentamicin
      d. Diazepam
      e. Sedatives
      f. Opiates
      g. Alcohol
      h. Neuroleptics
      i. Aspirin
      j. Nicotine
      k. Caffeine
  7. Cardiac
      a. Arrhythmia
      b. Hypertension
      c. Hypotension
      d. Poor cardiac output

E. Treatment
  1. Mild: Promethazine hydrochloride, 25 mg every 6 hours po as needed, or diazepam, 5 mg every 6 hours po as needed
  2. Moderate: Promethazine hydrochloride IV until stable, then promethazine by mouth or by rectal suppository
  3. Severe or with dehydration: IV fluids and parenteral phenothiazines; occasionally use supplemental diazepam or droperidol

V. FACIAL PARALYSIS WORK-UP AND TREATMENT
  A. History
    1. Gradual versus sudden onset
    2. Family history
    3. Pregnancy
    4. Head trauma
    5. Ear disease
    6. Parotid neoplasm
  B. Examination must include
    1. Otoscopy
    2. Hearing test, including tympanometry
    3. Eyes: Test tearing with Schirmer paper
    4. Mouth: Check tongue—chorda tympani is responsible for sense of taste on anterior two thirds of tongue and for submandibular gland salivary stimulation
    5. Face: Examination for muscle and nerve function; may need to test function electrically
    6. Neck: Check for parotid tumor
    7. Temporal bone tomography to rule out cerebellopontine angle tumor
  C. Treatment of Acute Paralysis
    1. Treat specific cause if known
    2. For idiopathic cases
      a. Partial paralysis: Observe
      b. Total paralysis with no electrical conduction: Consider total facial nerve decompression
    3. If the eye does not close or tearing is decreased, or both, treat eye to prevent corneal drying with eye drops during the day and moisture chamber at night
  D. Facial Rehabilitation
    1. Facial nerve graft
    2. Hypoglossal to facial nerve anastomosis
    3. Temporalis muscle sling

VI. NOSE
  A. Epistaxis
    1. Anterior bleeding site: identify by visual examination

    a. Hold cocaine-impregnated pledget against bleeding site
    b. Inject with lidocaine with 1% epinephrine
    c. Apply $\frac{1}{2}$-in gauze anterior nasal pack
  2. Posterior bleeding site
    a. Use 30-ml Foley balloon as a posterior pack
    b. Use $\frac{1}{2}$-in gauze as an anterior nasal pack
    c. Admit patient to hospital, apply O_2 mask, give minimal sedation or analgesia
  3. If bleeding continues, or if it recurs after removing pack at 3 to 4 days, then surgery (internal maxillary artery ligation and ethmoid artery ligation) should be performed

B. Sinusitis
  1. Symptoms
    a. Pain
    b. Pressure
    c. Elevated temperature
    d. Nasal discharge or postnasal drip
  2. Signs
    a. Pain elicited by tapping directly over sinus
    b. Elevated temperature
    c. Erythematous oropharynx
  3. Acute episodes are often associated with upper respiratory tract infections or episodes of acute allergic rhinitis
  4. Nasal endoscopy—ostiomeatal complex disease
  5. If chronic, sinus CT
  6. Treatment for acute sinusitis
    a. amoxicillin 250 mg
      1 p.o. tid for 10 to 14 days
    b. Decongestant prn
    c. Normal saline nasal douche: Dispense 120 ml of normal saline
      Three drops sniffed deeply into each nostril q4h and prn for stuffiness
  7. Treatment for chronic sinusitis
    a. antibiotics for 3 to 12 weeks
    b. Nasal evaluation
      i. cytology
      ii. IgE
      iii. endoscopy
      iv. sinus CT
    c. Appropriate allergic therapy
      i. antihistamine
      ii. environmental control

          iii. nasal steroids

          iv. desensitazation

          v. endoscopic sinus surgery

C. Nasal Obstruction
  1. Unilateral causes
     a. Foreign body
     b. Nasal polyp
     c. Nasal or nasal pharyngeal cancer
     d. Septal deviation
  2. Bilateral causes
     a. Nasal polyps
     b. Septal deviation
     c. Inflammatory rhinosinusitis
     d. Aging
  3. Treatment
     For all conditions mentioned except allergic rhinitis, surgery is required; patient should be referred to a head and neck surgeon
  4. Allergic rhinitis
     a. Environmental control
     b. Decongestant–antihistamine combination (one of the following):
        i. Actifed®, tid or qid
        ii. Dimetapp®, bid
        iii. Drixoral®, bid
        iv. Ornade®, bid
        v. Terfenadine® bid (H1 specific)
        vi. Astemizole® q.day (H1 specific)
     c. Intranasal steroids
     d. Cromolyn sodium
     e. If unsuccessful, refer the patient to an allergist for allergic testing and possible desensitization
D. Olfactory Dysfunction
  1. Causes
     a. Inflammatory rhinitis
     b. Trauma
     c. Postviral
     d. Toxin
     e. Congenital
     f. Psychiatric
     g. Alzheimer's disease
     h. Aging
  2. Evaluation
     a. Smell test
     b. Nasal cytology
     c. IgE and RAST screen
     d. Nasal endoscopy

      e. Sinus CT
      f. Consider trial of steroids
   3. Treatment
      a. Specific treatment for specific disease
      b. Smoke detectors, gas detectors, spoiled food patrol
      c. Taste rehabilitation

VII. THROAT (Oral Cavity, Oropharynx, Larynx, Hypopharynx, Esophagus, Trachea)
  A. Tonsillitis
    1. Symptoms
      a. Sore throat: usually severe; occasionally interferes with swallowing, rarely with breathing
      b. Elevated temperature: children, 103–105°F; adults, 101–103°F
      c. Patient feels sick
      d. No runny nose
    2. Signs
      a. Reddened tonsils, often with white lymphoid exudates
      b. Pharynx and nose are normal on examination
      c. Cervical lymph nodes often enlarged
      d. Elevated temperature
    3. Throat Culture: if positive, will show beta-hemolytic streptococcus, but unfortunately is positive only two thirds of the time; culture is often expensive and for both reasons can be limited to
      a. Patients with known valvular or rheumatic heart disease
      b. Immunosuppressed patients
      c. Patients who insist or whose parents insist on having a culture performed
    4. Treatment
      a. Adults: penicillin, 250 mg by mouth four times daily for 10 days
      b. Children: penicillin, 75 mg/kg/d in four equal doses, not to exceed 1 g/d
      c. Patients allergic to penicillin should be given erythromycin
    5. Indications for Surgery
      a. A single episode requiring hosptialization for dysphagia or dyspnea
      b. More than four episodes per year for at least 2 years, causing patient to miss 10 days of school or work annually
      c. Recurrent tonsillitis causing recurrent otitis media

B. Viral Pharyngitis
   1. Symptoms
      a. Sore throat
      b. Usually followed closely by runny nose
   2. Signs
      a. Diffuse pharyngitis including but not confined to tonsils
      b. Clear or purulent rhinitis; usually without significant cervical adenopathy
   3. Treatment: this is a viral disease and as such is not altered by antibiotic therapy. Decongestant–antihistamine combination therapy will diminish nasal symptoms. Antibiotics indicated only for purulent rhinitis, recurrent otitis media, or recurrent sinusitis. Tonsilectomy is also ineffective and is not indicated
C. Peritonsillar Abscess (PTA)
   1. Symptoms: severe sore throat, often unilateral, usually with significant dysphagia, temperature, elevation, and malaise
   2. Signs: unilateral protuberant tonsil, often with soft palate or uvular edema and occasionally with uvular deviation away from the involved side
   3. Diagnosis: made by anesthetizing the superior pole of tonsils and adjacent soft palate and then aspirating or incising and draining pus
   4. Culture and sensitivity tests and gram stain will often show mixed anaerobic infection
   5. Treatment Plan I
      a. Incision and drainage
      b. Hospitalization
      c. Intravenous fluids and penicillin, 2 million U IV every 6 hours until specific sensitivity tests results are known
      d. Antibiotics for 10 days; not necessarily IV for all 10 days
      e. Elective tonsillectomy 6 weeks after recovery
   6. Treatment Plan II
      a. Aspirate pus, confirming diagnosis and obtaining material for culture and sensitivity tests
      b. Admit patient to hospital and begin IV penicillin therapy
      c. Immediate tonsillectomy by head and neck surgeon
   7. Treatment Plan III
      a. Needle aspiration up to three times
      b. Oral antibiotics
      c. Follow-up prn

D. Differential Diagnosis for Sore Throat
  1. Beta-hemolytic streptococcal tonsillitis
  2. Viral pharyngitis
  3. Peritonsillar abscess
  4. Mononucleosis: positive mononucleosis spot test
  5. Gonococcal pharyngitis: positive sexual history and positive gonococcal culture
  6. Atypical infection, such as with *Mycobacterium, Treponema,* or *Candida:* diagnose by proper culture
  7. Recurrent herpes pharyngitis: diagnose by typical history
  8. Oropharyngeal neoplasm: Biopsy
  9. Allergic pharyngitis: often food allergy
  10. Smokers' and drinkers' pharyngitis
  11. Pharyngitis sicca: a condition seen in mouth breathers, especially in low-humidity conditions, or in elderly patients with atrophic mucosa and poor fluid intake. Also seen in patients after radiation therapy or in patients with Sjögren's syndrome

E. Oral Cavity Venereal Disease
  1. Gonorrhea: usually pharyngitis, diagnosed by positive sexual history and culture
  2. Syphilis: primary chancre, positive sexual history and culture, positive VDRL test
  3. Papilloma: Venereal warts, usually multiple; positive sexual history. Treat with cryotherapy, diathermy, or surgical excision
  4. Recurrent herpes pharyngitis: usually found in patients with venereal herpes; tends to recur during periods of stress. Physical findings show a few clear, fluid-filled vesicles in oropharynx

F. Globus Hysterius
  1. Symptoms: a feeling of fullness in throat, a lump in throat associated with swallowing, or tightness in throat
  2. Signs: normal results on head and neck examination
  3. Treatment: This is a psychologic response to some type of stress, almost always revealed by taking a careful history. Refer the patient for appropriate psychologic psychiatric counseling. *Do not order barium swallow*

G. Foreign Bodies in the Airway
  1. Occurs most commonly in the very young, usually 8 months to 3 or 4 years
  2. Symptoms
    a. Aphonia and acute respiratory obstruction when there is total airway obstruction
    b. Coughing with inspiratory or expiratory stridor breathing when there is partial obstruction

    3.   Treatment

        a. Total obstruction: use the Heimlich maneuver for young and old alike. If unsuccessful *emergeny cricothyrotomy is required*

        b. Partial obstruction: keep the patient quiet and transport to operating room for removal of the foreign body under anesthesia. Obtain cervical or chest X rays, or both, to localize the foreign body

H. Foreign Bodies in the Esophagus

    1.   Symptoms: choking while eating, often on a fish bone or chicken bone. Frequently hurts at first and then the pain subsides. If foreign body persists, signs of infection will begin to develop around three days later

    2.   Evaluation: includes careful history and soft tissue X rays; if these are not diagnostic, perform a barium swallow with cotton pledget soaked in barium

    3.   Treatment: if history or X rays give even a slight suspicion of a foreign body, rigid endoscopy under general anesthesia is required

I. Hoarseness: Voice changes resulting in breathy, rough, or coarse sound. Common causes include

    1.   Acute viral laryngitis: Often associated with upper respiratory infection; this is self-limiting and will disappear in 7 to 10 days, but patient should use voice sparingly

    2.   Vocal cord nodules: caused by voice abuse (usually screaming and yelling excessively), smoking, and sometimes endotracheal intubation. Diagnosis is made by mirror laryngoscopy; treat patient by ordering voice rest, speech therapy, and sometimes microlaryngoscopy with vocal cord stripping

    3.   Vocal cord paralysis: caused by trauma, laryngeal cancers, and occasionally superior mediastinal diseases or cardiac dilation affecting the left recurrent laryngeal nerve. Diagnosis is by mirror laryngoscopy and then by complete work-up to determine its pathogenesis. Treatment depends on the cause

    4.   Laryngeal cancer: usually found in middle-aged or older smokers. Diagnosis is by mirror laryngoscopy followed by direct laryngoscopy with biopsies. These tumors are treated primarily by head and neck surgeons

J. Acute Epiglottis (Supraglottitis)

    1.   Symptoms: acute respiratory distress, primarily inspiratory. Patient is toxic, prefers sitting up, and as symptoms progress develops increasing air hunger and inspiratory stridor

    2.   Signs: toxic, febrile child. Epiglottis swollen and red. Blood cultures reveal *Haemophilus influenzae*

3. Treatment: give IV dexamethasone and ampicillin. Give humidified air, oxygen, and racemic epinephrine by mask. Patients with mild cases can be observed in intensive care; if they begin to improve, will recover rapidly. Patients with severe cases are brought directly to the operating room with a head and neck surgeon and an anesthesiologist in attendance. If under anesthesia the patient can be intubated, that is sufficient. If not, emergency tracheostomy will be necessary. A 7- to 10-day course of ampicillin is necessary. Patient can be extubated after 48 to 72 hours or the tracheostomy tube can be removed after 3 to 4 days

VIII. NECK MASSES: DIFFERENTIAL DIAGNOSIS AND EVALUATION
   A. Congenital neck masses: occur predominantly between birth and 30 years of age
      1. Branchial cleft cyst: occurs often as an infected cyst; appears in the high lateral neck along the jugular vein
      2. Thyroglossal duct cyst: appears in the midline between the hyoid bone and sternal notch; often appears as an infected cyst
      3. Hemangioma and lymphangioma: these can appear anywhere in the head and neck and can be localized or extensive
   B. Traumatic Neck Masses
      1. Arteriovenous fistula secondary to penetrating trauma; diagnose by history and bruit
      2. Laryngocele: usually found on left side in patients playing a musical instrument such as bugle or trumpet; diagnosis is by history, physical examination, and laryngography
   C. Inflammatory Neck Masses
      1. Viral lymphadenitis: common in children with viral upper respiratory tract infection; lymph nodes are multiple, soft, mobile, and rarely larger than 2 cm across
      2. Bacterial abscess: may be secondary to direct penetrating injury, abscessed viral lymph node, or a primary infective process in the head and neck, such as a dental abscess. Patient is usually sick, often toxic. Mass can be firm if under pressure or fluctuant. Aspiration of pus is diagnostic. Organisms are often anaerobic. Treat by surgical drainage
      3. Other common infectious causes
         a. Tuberculosis
         b. Coccidiomycosis
         c. Mycobacterium
         d. Syphilis
         e. Cat-scratch fever

    4. Ludwig's angina: an abscess under the floor of the mouth that presents under the chin. The lesion is of particular concern because it may push the tongue posteriorly, thereby causing respiratory obstruction.

    5. AIDS: Various HIV-related illnesses can present as a cervical mass; biopsy is often required

  D. Neoplastic Neck Masses

    1. Lymphoma: Masses are often multiple and can be unilateral or bilateral; they can be large (up to 10 cm) or small, and are usually soft and mobile

    2. Epidermoid carcinoma: a tumor found in the fourth decade of life and later. It results from effects of tobacco use that are enhanced by alcohol intake. The cervical disease is metastatic from a primary lesion somewhere in the mucosa of the upper aerodigestive tract. The neck mass can be large. It is usually hard and may be fixed. Diagnosis is by discovery and biopsy of the primary lesion

    3. Metastatic cancers from the chest and abdomen: spread is usually via the lymphatics and the mass is in the supraclavicular fossa. Full work-up and then biopsy are indicated

    4. Thyroid Cancer: thyroid mass or cervical metastases may be the initial presenting feature. Careful examination should reveal the thyroid primary tumor. Diagnosis is by FNA; ultrasound, thyroid scan, or open biopsy

    5. Other Tumors: A variety of other tumors, such as melanoma, sarcoma, plasmacytoma, and adenocarcinoma, may present in the neck. If one of these is suspected, diagnosis is made by a full evaluation and finally a biopsy

  E. Metabolic Neck Masses

    1. Graves' disease

    2. Goiter

    3. Parathyroid Tumors

All of these should be obvious; the Graves' tumor and parathyroid tumors should have endocrine manifestations—a full evaluation is indicated

IX. HEAD AND NECK CANCER

  A. Salivary Gland Cancer

    1. Constitutes about 3% of head and neck tumors; 80% involve the parotid gland. Of parotid tumors, 80% are benign (60% are pleomorphic adenomas), whereas 50% of submandibular and sublingual tumors are malignant

    2. Benign tumors include pleomorphic adenoma, papillary cystadenoma lymphomatosum (Warthin's tumor), and oncocytoma. Malignant tumors include muco-

epidermoid carcinoma, adenoid cystic carcinoma, adenocarcinoma, epidermoid carcinoma, and undifferentiated carcinoma

B. Epidermoid Carcinoma of the Mucosal Surfaces of the Upper Aerodigestive Tract
   1. Includes tumors of the nasal cavity and paranasal sinuses, oral cavity, oropharynx, nasopharynx, hypopharynx, larynx, and cervical esophagus
   2. These tumors are induced by tobacco; the tobacco effect is greatly enhanced by alcohol intake
   3. Symptoms
      a. Pain
      b. Hoarseness
      c. Obstruction to respiration or swallowing
      d. Weight loss
      e. Malaise or neck masses
   4. Evaluation: includes a complete history and physical examination, biopsy of the primary site, complete blood cell count, urinalysis, determinations of creatinine, blood urea nitrogen, serum glutamic pyruvic transaminase, alkaline phosphatase, and bilirubin (total and direct) levels, and chest X ray
   5. Direct laryngoscopy and esophagoscopy should be performed to evaluate the extent of the cancer fully, to rule out second primary lesions, and to discover the primary lesion in patients presenting with neck masses
   6. Treatment: includes surgery and radiation therapy, often in combination; chemotherapy is only adjunctive or palliative
C. Thyroid Cancer
   1. Includes papillary carcinoma, follicular carcinoma, mixed papillary and follicular carcinoma, Hürthle cell carcinoma, medullary carcinoma, and anaplastic carcinoma
   2. Patient usually presents with an asymptomatic thyroid or cervical mass
   3. History may include previously irradiation to neck
   4. Evaluation includes T_4, T_3, TSH and thyroid scan, ultrasound and/or FNA
   5. Diagnosis is by observation to see if the mass is enlarging, FNA, and finally lobectomy
   6. Treatment: Total thyroidectomy and excision of all cervical metastases; patient should be maintained on thyroid extract after surgery
D. Skin Cancer
   1. Basal cell tumors
      a. Diagnosis is by inspection and punch biopsy

     b. Treatment: includes curettage and desiccation for superficial lesions and surgery for large and deeper lesions

     c. Recurrent basal cell tumors and sclerosing basal cell tumors should be treated with microscopically controlled excision called Mohs' chemosurgery

2. Epidermoid cancer

     a. Diagnosis is by inspection and punch biopsy

     b. Treatment: surgical excision

     c. Recurrent large or invasive epidermoid cancers should be removed with microscopically controlled excision

3. Melanoma

     a. Diagnosis is by inspection and *excisional* biopsy

     b. Staging by depth of invasion is important

     c. Treatment: wide surgical excision with neck dissection only if metastasis exists

     d. Postoperative radiation therapy is indicated for advanced lesions

     e. Immunologic chemotherapy consultations should always be requested

X. MAXILLOFACIAL TRAUMA

A. Evaluation

1. For soft tissue trauma, evaluate

     a. Skin

     b. Muscle

     c. Nerves

     d. Major vessels

     e. Mucosa

2. For trauma to facial bones, evaluate by observations, palpation, and X rays

3. Eyes: check vision and extraocular eye movements

4. Ears: test hearing and look for hemotympanum

5. Nose: look for bleeding and cerebrospinal fluid leak

6. Mouth: Examine teeth and occlusion

B. X rays if bony trauma is suspected

1. Facial series

     a. Posteroanterior

     b. Waters

     c. Submental vertical

     d. Lateral

2. Mandibular series

     a. Posteroanterior

     b. Right and left oblique

     c. Transorbital view of condyle and/or

     d. Panorex

    3. CT scan

    4. Nose: Nasal X rays are not indicated

C. Treatment

    1. Soft tissue

       a. Clean

       b. Debride dead tissues

       c. Stop bleeding

       d. Repair nerves

       e. Repair muscles

       f. Close subcutaneous tissue and skin

    2. Bone: bony fractures are repaired if functional or cosmetic defects exist; common fractures include

       a. Trimalar (Zygoma or malar, or both) fracture

          i. Elevate zygomatic arch

         ii. Reduce fracture to restore normal facial contour

       b. Orbital floor fracture

          i. Observe for enophthalmos

         ii. Observe for diplopia with muscular entrapment

        iii. Explore and repair only when diplopia with entrapment or enophthalmos is present

       c. Nasal fracture

          i. Reduce for cosmetic reasons

         ii. Look for and treat septal hematoma

       d. Maxillary fractures: all fractures (often called LeFort) must be repaired to restore normal dental occlusion; all patients receive arch bars with interdental fixation

       e. Mandibular fracture: Reduce fracture, place arch bars with interdental fixation

IX. LARYNX: all laryngeal fractures require indirect or direct laryngoscopy by head and neck surgeons. Fractures are opened and reduced. The larynx or trachea is then stented.

Suggested Readings

GENERAL TEXTBOOKS

Cummings C, et al, eds. Otolaryngology—Head and neck surgery. 2d ed. St. Louis: CV Mosby; 1991.
An excellent four-volume text, used by many head and neck surgery residents as their primary textbook.
Paparella MM, Shumrick OA. Otolaryngology. 3d ed. Philadelphia: WB Saunders; 1990.
A textbook also used by many residents. Either of these first two major works should supply substantial background information.
Lee KJ. Textbook of otolaryngology—Head and neck surgery. New York: Elsevier; 1989.
A shorter textbook, extremely concise and yet complete, primarily designed as a board review text; many head and neck surgery residents read this in preparation for their boards. Contains a lot of data, but lacks basic science explanation and depth.

ANATOMY

Hollingshead WH. Textbook of anatomy, Vol. 1—The head and neck. 4th ed. Philadelphia: Harper and Row; 1985.
The most commonly used textbook of head and neck anatomy. Although it contains some pictures, it is primarily descriptive. More thorough than Grays and Grants.
Pernkopf E. Anatomy of topographic and applied human anatomy. 3d ed. Baltimore: Urban and Schwarzenberg; 1989.
A premiere color atlas, probably even more thorough then Grant's Atlas of Anatomy. Each picture is a work of art.

SURGICAL ATLASES AND TEXTS

Montgomery WW. Surgery of the upper respiratory system, Vols. 1 and 2. 2d ed. Philadelphia: Lea & Febiger; 1989.
An excellent atlas of upper respiratory tract surgery, including most of the important operations on the upper aerodigestive system, including nose, oral cavity, pharynx, larynx, and cervical esophagus.

Lore JM. Atlas of head and neck surgery. 3d ed. Philadelphia: WB Saunders; 1988.
An excellent surgical text.
Glasscock ME, Shambaugh GE, Surgery of the ear. 4th ed. Philadelphia: WB Saunders; 1990.
There are many otologic surgery atlases. This one is excellent.
Schuknecht HS. Pathology of the ear. Cambridge: Harvard University Press; 1974.
A masterful otologic text.

FACIAL PLASTIC AND RECONSTRUCTIVE SURGERY

Mathog R. Maxillofacial trauma. Baltimore: Williams & Wilkins; 1991.
A complete review of the evaluation and management of maxillofacial trauma.
Rees TD, Asethetic plastic surgery, Vols. I and II. Philadelphia: WB Saunders; 1980.
One of the better textbooks on today's cosmetic facial surgery.
Sheen JH. Aesthetic rhinoplasty. 2d ed. St. Louis: Mosby; 1987.
A superlative text on rhinoplasty. It is advanced but it is well illustrated.

HISTOLOGY

Batsakis. Tumors of the head and neck: Clinical and pathological considerations. Baltimore: Williams & Wilkins; 1979.
The classic on histology of head and neck tumors.

HEAD AND NECK CANCER

Suen JY, Myers EN. Cancer of the head and neck. 2d ed. New York: Churchill Livingstone; 1989.
Rice OH, Spiro RH. Current concepts in head and neck cancer. American Cancer Society; 1989.
There are many excellent head and neck cancer textbooks. These are two current examples.

COLOR ATLASES

Becker W. Atlas of otorhinolaryngology and bronchoesophagology. Philadelphia: WB Saunders; 1969.
Kleinsasser O. Microlaryngoscopy and endolaryngeal microsurgery. Philadelphia: WB Saunders; 1968.
Colby RA, Robinson HBG. Color atlas of oral pathology. 5th ed. Philadelphia: Lippincott; 1990.
These three atlases show pictures of areas and diseases that are rarely shown and, hence, are excellent sources for the interested reader.

VIDEOTAPES

Head and Neck Surgery for Medical Students. An 8-hour series showing head and neck examination, aspects of head and neck surgery, facial plastic and reconstructive surgery, head and neck cancer, and the techniques of emergency tracheostomy and epistaxis. Distributed by the American Academy of Otolaryngology—Head and Neck Surgery, 1 Prince Street, Alexandria, VA 22314.

Medical Journals in Otolaryngology—Head and Neck Surgery

Laryngoscope, The Triological Foundation, Inc., St. Louis.

Archives of Otolaryngology—Head and Neck Surgery, American Medical Association, Chicago.

Head and Neck Surgery, John Wiley & Sons, New York.

Journal of Otolaryngology—Head and Neck Surgery, Mosby-Year Book, St. Louis.

The above journals are the broadest publications in otolaryngology—head and neck surgery. The journals that follow are specialized.

American Journal of Rhinology, OceanSide Publications, Inc., Providence, RI.

Journal of Plastic and Reconstructive Surgery, Williams & Wilkins, Baltimore.

Journal of Voice Disorders, Raven Press, New York.

American Journal of Otology, B.C. Decker, Inc., Hamilton, Ontario.

Index

Page numbers followed by *f* indicate illustrations.
Page numbers followed by *t* indicate tables.